When A Document Takes Affect	If person is unavailable but otherwise competent	If person is unable to make decisions for self but not permanently unconscious or terminally ill	If person is permanently unconscious or terminally ill	Upon death
Will	NO	NO	NO	YES
Durable Power of Attorney (POA)	YES	YES	YES	NO
Living Will	n/a	NO	YES	NO
Health Care POA	n/a	YES	YES	NO

- Beware of SCAMS and undue influence

Memorial –
- Tuesdays with Morrie (book)
- Obituary & funeral considerations
- Surviving spouse

Emotional / Relational –
- Caregiver vs. care receiver perspective
- Person vs. circumstances
- Seek support & be supportive
- Don't squander the words I Love You

I've Learned – Chapter 10, p. 242-243

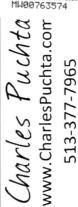

Charles Puchta
www.CharlesPuchta.com
513-377-7965

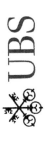

AGING & CAREGIVING – (4/26/13)

Desired Outcome –

1. Provoke thought about age-related considerations
2. Get conversations started

What is "Normal" Aging to You? Considering aspects that are most important may help you:

1. Understand values, personal beliefs and ideals related to the aging process.
2. Determine health goals and priorities for the later years of life.
3. Communicate personal preferences regarding self-care and the provision of care.

Common Challenges – The five 'In' words – Chapter 1, p. 34-35

Lifestyle –

- Diagnosis vs. prognosis
- 10 Considerations – 2nd Chapter, p. 47-48
- Daily living activities
  1. ADLs – Basic self-care (personal care)
  2. IADLs – Complex living skills (independent living)
- Consider aging parent / care receiver preferences

Administration –

- Financial, insurance and legal considerations

CAREGIVING

Ready or Not

CAREGIVING

Ready or Not

Essential Information and Insight for Boomers

CHARLES PUCHTA

Published by:

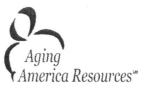

Cincinnati

Inquires should be addressed to
Aging America Resources
11611 Kosine Lane, Suite 105
Loveland, OH 45140-1912

ISBN: 978-0-9722104-7-8

Printed in the United States of America

Library of Congress Control Number: Pending

To my wife, Karen, and our daughters Josie, Ellie and
Abbie. I love you more than words can express.
Thanks for your love, support and encouragement.

Also, to Dean Andrea Lindell, Evelyn Fitzwater
and Cindy Cook of the University of Cincinnati
College of Nursing. Your commitment to ensuring
quality and dignified care is an inspiration to me.

This book is dedicated to the many family and
professional caregivers who selflessly give their time,
talent and treasures for the benefit of others.

In memory of my parents:
Charles G. Puchta   1918 – 1997
Jean G. Puchta   1931 – 2001

DISCLAIMER: *THIS BOOK PROVIDES INSIGHT AND
ENCOURAGMENT, NOT ABSOLUTES OR ANSWERS.*

Contact your financial, legal, medical and spiritual
advisors for advice specific to your situation.
Our resources are intended to complement,
not substitute, professional advice.

embrace ■ ■ ■
caregiving^{SM}

Greetings,

    CAREGIVING Ready or Not is one in a series of books I have written to help boomers and older adults who are caring for a parent, spouse, relative or friend. The purpose of this book is to help caregivers anticipate, understand and address the many issues they are likely to face as a result of aging, illness or injury. This book reflects my personal and professional experience, extensive literature reviews and findings from research, along with the stories of hundreds of people who have shared their experiences and frustrations for the benefit of others.

    This book cuts through the clutter and confusion and offers clear and unbiased information and insight to help caregivers and care receivers make informed decisions. Throughout the book, I provide practical knowledge, tools and tips that you and your family can immediately begin applying. I also offer thought-provoking and actionable perspectives to help you along your journey ahead – *Ready or Not.*

    Many people believe that *"Information is power."* I disagree. Rather, I believe that *"Information applied is power."* After all, if you can't *do* something with your new knowledge and act on it, what good is it? My hope is that I have effectively addressed the subject matter in a way that equips, empowers and encourages you to confidently apply this information and make wise choices.

    As you begin working your way through *CAREGIVING Ready or Not,* I encourage you to get a pen, highlight sections and write notes in the margins. There is also a space at the end of every section for you to note key learnings and action items. For information about other resources I have written or offer, please visit www.Caregiving.CC and www.Puchta.CC. You may also enjoy and find my other books to be helpful. *CARE for One Another* offers a Christian perspective on caregiving and explores biblical caregiving principles. My other book *Engaging While AGING* offers helpful information and insight to help Baby Boomers and mature adults address the many significant life decisions and transitions they are likely to encounter as they age. I wish you the best along your journey – *Ready or Not.*

May God bless you!

Charles Puchta

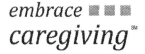

Embrace caregiving is a service mark of Aging America Resources and is the brand under which we offer our products and services.

Aging America Resources is a 501(c)(3) nonprofit organization.

About the Author

Charles Puchta is founder and principal of Aging America Resources (www.Caregiving.CC), Director of the Center for Aging with Dignity (www.SAFEafter60.CC) at the University of Cincinnati College of Nursing and an adjunct instructor for the UC School of Health Services. Puchta is a Certified Senior Advisor, an award-winning author and a nationally recognized authority, advisor, advocate, and speaker on the subject of aging and caregiving.

He has devoted his life to helping individuals, families and professionals anticipate, understand and address the many challenges brought about by aging and illness. His distinctive gift is his ability to take complex subject matter, distill it and communicate it in a way that makes sense to the audience.

Puchta has written numerous books, small group curriculums and other resources addressing aging, health concerns and caregiving issues. He works with organizations across the country, helping them formulate and implement programs to support the care needs of older adults and caregivers. For more information, visit www.Puchta.CC.

Puchta lives in Loveland, Ohio, with his wife, three daughters and two dogs. A favorite saying, and one that reflects his career and calling is, *"To love what you do and feel that it matters – how could anything be more fun?"*

In addition to the fun he has pursuing his passion, Puchta believes that caregiving should be fulfilling and rewarding for both the care receiver and caregiver. He hopes, and is confident that, this book will provide you with the perspectives and practical insight you need to make a difference in the lives of the people with whom you interact.

Comments

Chuck, God has brought me your book at yet another huge crossroad in decisions my family is needing to make concerning my parents. I am absolutely amazed (but shouldn't be!) that just when I had once again thought I was losing my mind, He dropped your book in my lap. Somehow my sisters and I have muddled through about seven years that have seemed like an endless maze of decisions, crises, unexpected events, and family dynamics. And each time we thought things might be settling down a bit--sorry but nope! The other shoe always drops. Or as a good friend of mine says, *"If it's not one thing, it's your mother."*

When life gets particularly stressful, I have a hard time sitting down long enough to read a how-to that might actually alleviate my stress! Wow! You've nailed it. Your approach is right on-target. Your style of talking straight to issues and concerns of Boomers is perfect. You speak our language!

Your book is a wonderful combination of educating, coaching, encouraging, and practical help. *(I was skeptical that you could accomplish all that in one book on this topic, since many authors try, but fall short in one area or another.)* As I am reading it, I feel refreshed and empowered, not overwhelmed and burdened with too much information. Boomers like me who are in the midst of the battle, need this type of focused, clear-cut, orderly and digestible book. Your expertise and knowledge are impressive, and you have a humble, clear way of getting that information into a reader's hands.

After reading first book years ago and realizing you were a goldmine I was going to need some day, I gave your book to a friend in the midst of caregiving crisis. While I know it was helpful to her, I am kicking myself that I missed all the good info while we were living the first part of our journey, I still have to trust that God's timing is perfect....He gave me His wisdom through you at the beginning of the process, and now He's brought me full circle as my mom and dad are both reaching the end stages of their illnesses.

Your book is a true blessing, and I thank you from the bottom of my heart for allowing God to use you as His special agent in a time of need.

Margaret Behlert

Charles, you have masterfully presented practical and actionable information about a very complex subject. *CAREGIVING Ready or Not* accurately, clearly and fairly portrays the realities Baby Boomers are sure to encounter caring for aging parents. As I read your book I found myself saying "yes" over and over again as you hit all the salient points every caregiver needs to know and understand. The way you incorporated your personal story, quotes and poems adds a dimension that caregivers long for.

As a nurse specializing in gerontology, and one who has been on the care receiving side, I especially appreciate your respectful attitude toward older adults. All too often adult children try to take over thinking they know what is best. Then when they become stressed and frustrated because their aging parents are not receptive, they wonder why. The way you explain the partnership that is essential to caring relationships is brilliant.

Caregivers desperately need to see life through the lens of the care receiver as doing so can bring understanding and compassion to their gestures and interactions. Simply put, your book is a must read for anyone taking on the caregiver role, regardless of whether they think they are Ready or Not.

Evelyn Fitzwater, DSN, RN

Contents

Introduction

CAREGIVING Ready or Not provides the foundational understanding that caregivers so desperately need. With all the talk about the frustrations and challenges caregivers face on a day-to-day basis, I have my own theory about caregiver stress. I believe that caregivers often bring much of the stress on themselves by wanting to control the situation. My advice for all caregivers, whether family or professional, is to include the care receivers in their planning, decisions and daily activities. Rather than trying to force people to do what we think is best, caregivers will have a much more rewarding experience if they make plans and set goals *with* the care receivers, not *for* them.

Sure, the relationship dynamics between you and your loved ones change with due to age-related limitations and illness. And yes, you are certainly and rightfully going to get frustrated from time to time as the same story or question is repeated over and over, or the personal care requirements become physically draining. However, as long as the care receiver is of sound mind and able to make decisions on his or her own, he or she has the right to do so.

The journey I take you through in this book starts with helping you make sense of your situation, discovering your roles and responsibilities, exploring the aging process and seeing life through the lens of a care receiver. Midway through the book I delve deeper into practical and purposeful caregiving, address discussions, decisions and dynamics along with conflict communication strategies. Then I wrap things up addressing loss and grieving, sharing end-of-life considerations, and ideas to help ensure lasting memories. These are all topics caregivers need to know and understand, as doing so will help them engage in more meaningful and supportive ways.

As caregivers there is a natural tendency to want to jump into the tasks and start doing things. My recommendation is not to overlook the importance of relationship. Often, the best present we can provide to our loved ones is our presence. For caregivers who are long distance, your regular communication, whether over the phone or via the internet, is equally important. I wholeheartedly believe that caregivers need to realize and understand the human *being* part before becoming immersed as a human *doing*.

Engaging While AGING is a follow-up to this book. In this book I address important considerations and transitions that older adults need to be prepared for, and baby boomers should begin considering, assuming they have not already done so. I begin this book with a look at the affects of aging, ways to age well and how to minimize safety risks. Knowing that older adults and people with chronic and life-threatening illnesses are likely to encounter many important and difficult decisions, I address the issues they are likely to face, explain the common concerns, explain the various options that might be available and offer advice to help people avoid surprises.

In this book I cover topics such as driving/transportation, and living environments and care arrangement. I offer insight and share information everyone needs to know about advance directives, legal and financial planning. I address government services, insurance options, Hospice care, funeral planning, the handling of personal belongings, and more. The reason *Engaging* is the word in the title is because baby boomers and older adults need to purposefully give consideration and deliberately make choices. When life becomes increasingly challenging due to age-related limitations and diseases, I find that maintaining control over life becomes increasingly important. The best way to maintain control is to give serious consideration to the issues you are likely to encounter, understand the options, determine your preferences and express your wishes to those who could be called upon to provide support. *Engaging While AGING* steps you through the issues and options, and offers considerations to help you determine what might be best based on your particular situation. In addition, I share insightful perspectives you are not likely to hear from family advisors and friends.

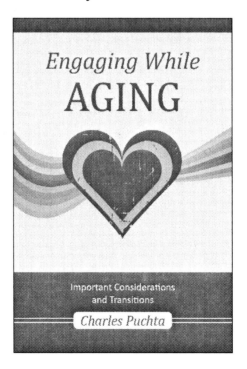

Available February '10 at www.Caregiving.CC

Introduction

"Love is more than a noun -- it is a verb;
it is more than a feeling -- it is caring,
sharing, helping, sacrificing."
– William Arthur Ward

1.

Making Sense of the Situation

Caregiving has quickly become an expected life event, just like getting married, having children, working and retiring. If you are not already providing care or support for a family member or friend, chances are you will at some time during your life. I hope that this book becomes a trusted and often-referenced resource. Throughout the book, I share information, insight and encouragement to help you along your journey so you can make the most of each day. I wish you the best as you make a difference in the lives of the people you love and that may have shown you similar kindness through the years.

A well-known quote by former First Lady Rosalynn Carter sums up the reality that we will all have our turn in the care process. *"There are only four kinds of people in the world:*

- *Those who have been caregivers.*
- *Those who currently are caregivers.*
- *Those who will be caregivers.*
- *Those who will need caregivers."* [1]

At sometime during our lives, 80% of Americans will be called upon to provide long-term care to parents, other family members or friends. The value of the care they provided is significant as loved ones will need assistance with daily living activities, care needs and social supports because of chronic illnesses and disabilities, many of which are age-related.[2]

The following are a few statistics about caregiving you might find interesting:

- Approximately 71% of baby boomers have at least one living parent. [3]
- 34 million adults (16% of the population) provide care to adults older than 50. [4, 5]
- 8.9 million caregivers (20% of adult caregivers) care for someone older than 50 who has dementia. [6]
- Approximately 40% of caregivers are adult children caring for their elderly parents. [7]
- Nearly 25% of caregivers are age 65 or older and provide care for a spouse. [8]
- An estimated third of all informal caregivers are employed full-time elsewhere. [9]
- Nearly 50% of caregivers provide fewer than eight hours of care per week, while an estimated 20% provide more than 40 hours of care per week. [10]
- Just over 65% of caregivers live with the care recipient or live within 20 minutes, whereas 15% of caregivers live an hour or more away. [11]
- Approximately 25% of care recipients live with the caregiver and 15% of caregivers live more than an hour from the care recipient. [12]

For additional facts and stats on caregiving, refer to the report *Caregiving in the U.S.* available at www.caregiving.org/data/04finalreport.pdf or visit the Caregiver Statistics page on the National Family Caregivers Association website at www.thefamilycaregiver.org.

For many people, it is a crisis situation that turns everyday life upside down and forces the realization that care and support are necessary. People often consider it a crisis when a loved one is unexpectedly hospitalized, diagnosed with a life-changing or a life-threatening disease or injured from a fall or accident. For others, caregiving may begin with a kind gesture, only to have the amount of involvement and responsibility increase over time. Kind gestures often include preparing the occasional meal, providing a ride to an appointment, helping to sort medications or lending a hand around the house.

Regardless of your situation or how it becomes apparent, many caregivers expect to be needed on a part-time basis, but the involvement may quickly become full-time. In situations where obligations to family, work and community limit your ability to provide the level of care a parent or other relative might need, you may find it necessary to supplement *informal* care, which is unpaid and provided by a family member, friend or neighbor, with *formal* care, which is provided by a paid and trained professional.

While each caregiving situation differs, most of the struggles individuals and families encounter are predictable. From the stories I have heard and the evidence I have seen, it appears that the challenges caregivers face are typically due to the lack of any of the following:

- Availability or participation of family because of work, family and community obligations, or living out of town.
- Agreement or cooperation from family members.
- Financial resources and affordability of needed services.
- Knowledge and confidence to take appropriate measures to provide for the safety, wellbeing and health of others.

Common Starting Points

For most people reading this book, one of three things has likely happened:

1. A life-changing event has occurred (e.g., illness, injury, hospitalization, or death).

2. You have come to realize or accept something that, up to this point, was not evident.

3. You are being proactive and want to be prepared for the future.

Examples of these starting points include:

1. Life-changing events:
   - Diagnosis of a chronic debilitating disease (e.g., Alzheimer's, arthritis, osteoporosis, Parkinson's).
   - Diagnosis of a terminal illness (e.g., cancer).
   - Medical emergency (e.g., heart attack, stroke).
   - Medication regimen requires the support of others.
   - Weekly doctor visits become necessary.
   - Oxygen or other support system becomes required.
   - Walker, wheelchair or other assistive device becomes necessary.
   - Hospitalization of one parent leaves the second parent home alone.

2. Realization on your part:
   - Noticeable change in functional capabilities.
   - Noticeable change in cognitive state.
   - Noticeable change in activity level.

- Realization that daily tasks are becoming more difficult and time-consuming (e.g., getting dressed, preparing a meal, balancing the checkbook).
- Apprehension to try new things or venture outside familiar territory.

3. Planning ahead: People often try to address a specific issue or topic such as:
- Knowing what signs to look for that may suggest physical and mental functional challenges.
- Understanding the various living environments and care options so that you are prepared if, and when, a change may be necessary.
- Ensuring that personal legal documents (e.g., Advance Directives, Will) are executed and up-to-date.
- Understanding one's wishes and expectations of family members.
- Developing a financial or retirement plan.
- Evaluating insurance coverage options (e.g., supplemental health, long-term care).
- Creating a legacy of memories while still possible.

The role of caregiver can be quite different based on the pattern of onset, the course of an illness, the degree of functional limitations or incapacitation and the expected outcome of any treatment. Also, the demands of a caregiver will differ based on the trajectory of an illness. For example, some conditions are progressive, whereas others may be constant or episodic.

Regardless of the challenges you are currently facing or which categories above represent your situation, know that you are not alone. There are many wonderful people, organizations and resources that can help you along your journey. In addition to friends and family, you might turn to people who have been down the road before and have dealt with a similar situation. Also, contact the appropriate national organization(s) (e.g., Alzheimer's Association, American Heart Association, National Stroke Association) for information and guidance.

Do You Consider Yourself A Caregiver?

An important first step for many people is to acknowledge that they are caregivers. Only then do they tend to reach out for the information, guidance and support that caregivers desperately need. As caregivers, we need knowledge, skills and confidence to effectively provide compassionate care. We also need to pursue lifestyle choices and behaviors that enhance health and quality of life.

Many people never consider themselves to be a caregiver. Instead, they view the support they provide as something a son, daughter, relative or friend naturally does. Another reason why people may not view themselves as caregivers is that it requires them to acknowledge that a loved one faces functional limitations and requires assistance – something many people would rather deny. Regardless of how you and your siblings envision your roles and responsibilities, your involvement can help aging or ill loved ones maintain their dignity and independence, and maximize their quality of life.

A favorite quote of mine is:

"A test of a people is how it behaves toward the old. It is easy to love children. Even tyrants and dictators make a point of being fond of children. But the affection and care for the old, the incurable, the helpless are the true gold mines of a culture."

> Abraham Joshua Heschel (1907-1972)
> Renowned educator, philosopher, rabbi
> and author

I wholeheartedly believe that caregivers are the true gold mines of a culture. Providing care and support for family and friends is a choice we make, a responsibility we accept and a gift that we give and receive. I find that because of the personal and private nature of health-related problems, many older adults and those with a chronic illness often overlook limitations, bottle up emotions and avoid talking about their situation. This can lead to caregivers isolating themselves and making things harder than they need to be.

While you may feel like you are alone, it is far from the truth. Family members are the predominate providers of long-term care. According to an AARP report entitled *Valuing the Invaluable: The Economic Value of Family Caregiving, 2008 Update*, there are more than 50 million people who served in a caregiving capacity at some time in 2007 with approximately 34 million providing care at any given time. These family members and friends are providing an estimated $375 billion worth of *free* services a year for loved ones who are aging, chronically ill or disabled. To arrive at the value, it is assumed that the services family caregivers provide for free would cost $10 per hour if paid.[13] While the cost of caregiving services varies across the county, if you work with a home care agency, you can expect to pay a minimum of $18-$20 per hour. One advantage of working with professional caregivers is that agencies provide training, conduct background checks, oversee the caregivers, handle the filings for Workers' Compensation, taxes and more.

There are many different definitions of caregiving. A few of my favorites include:

- *"A caregiver is anyone who provides assistance to someone else that is in some degree incapacitated and needs help."*
  – Family Caregiver Alliance (www.Caregiver.org) [14]

- *"A family caregiver is one who takes on the responsibility of caring for a friend or loved one who can no longer care for themselves, either due to mental, emotional or physical challenges."*

  – Gary Barg, founder of Caregiver Media Group (www.Caregiver.com) [15]

- *"[Family] Caregivers are those unpaid family members, friends and volunteers who provide care and assistance to people who are either chronically ill or disabled."*

  – Suzanne Mintz, President – National Family Caregivers Association (www.NFCAcares.org) [16]

Some organizations suggest that people cross over into the caregiver role once they consistently spend a certain number of hours a week in a capacity where they are providing care or support. Whether the number is 2 hours or 12 hours, the point remains the same; it is important for people to recognize themselves as caregivers.

Something I have said for years is that most *"caregivers do the best they do not know how to do"*. That is because they have never served as a caregiver before. If you have never done something before you cannot give it your best because you do not have a best. For example, when we say *"give it your best"* to kids before a sports competition, what is implied is that they are going to apply the skills and abilities they have developed from their coaches, practices, scrimmages and more.

With caregiving, reaching out to others is seeking information, guidance and support is critical. In addition to not knowing what to expect, what options might be available, and how to work through tough issues and make informed decisions, family dynamics often present unexpected challenging situations.

Taking Responsibility

Let's face it; family relationships can be complicated. Aging is something many people would rather deny, and the U.S. health care system is complex, specialized and difficult to navigate. Caregiving is full of unexpected twists, turns and turmoil. While there are no absolutes or answers, there is power in perspectives from people who understand your challenges and have been down the road before.

Long gone are the days that the family doctor directs the care process and proactively shares with us information we need to know now and what to expect in the future. Likewise, we cannot expect those we turn to for direction and support to provide us with what we need, when we need it. As a result, Americans must take increased responsibility for their wellness choices and their care.

When age-related health concerns become noticeable, or a loved one is diagnosed with a medical condition, a common reaction of caregivers is to search for information to become familiar with the condition or disease. From weekly magazines and tabloids, to infomercials and the Internet, there is no shortage of information and advice. *"The challenge these days is to find trustworthy medical information amid all the profit-driven, misleading, or just plain erroneous stuff on the Net."* [17]

Contrary to popular opinion and what is often reported in the media, a URL ending in .org does *not* mean the information is provided by a nonprofit organization or that it is credible. For example, the following information was recently reported in an article entitled *The 'Net: A Tangled Web of Health Information. "One good basic piece of advice is to stick to sites ending in '.edu,' '.gov' or '.org,'" Don Powell, president and CEO of the American Institute for Preventive Medicine, said.* [18] He indicated .edu websites are run by schools, .gov websites by government agencies, and .org websites by nonprofit organizations, whereas .com websites are commercial and would be likely to provide biased information.

Regardless of whether someone knows Dr. Powell, I can image that based on his affiliation, many people reading the article would think this information is accurate and credible. Unfortunately, the information is factually incorrect. Anyone can purchase a domain name ending in .org. As the screen shot from GoDaddy.com indicates, anyone willing to pay the price can buy a URL ending in .org, not just non-profit organizations.

When seeking information, use the Internet with caution! Consider the motivation of the person or entity offering the information. For example,

- Whom or what is the source of the information?
- Is it based on credible research?
- Is the person or entity sponsoring the Web site likely to be impartial?
- Is the Web site trying to convince you to buy something?
- Does the Web site feature advertising in prominent places?

A friend once made a profound statement that is worth repeating. When a parent is diagnosed with a disease, *"There should be a mandatory 30-day waiting period before anyone is allowed to go to the Internet to look for information about the disease."* Why? Because, the average person will find more information than he or she can ever comprehend and, all too often, the worst possible scenarios are presented. As such, people often become overwhelmed and may focus on inappropriate information. As you know, there is good information, as well as junk, on the Internet – *buyer (reader) beware*.

Recognizing the challenge of finding credible information, I recommend a free resource entitled *Getting Started* that is available at www.Caregiving.CC – click on *Articles* and then *Getting Started*. This document provides a list of credible agencies and organizations offering information about medical conditions, prescription drugs, aging and caregiving, government programs and services and more.

Family & Professional Caregivers

Family caregivers, also referred to as informal caregivers, traditionally have been unpaid family members, friends or neighbors who provide care on either a part-time or full-time basis. According to a Wall Street Journal article entitled *Wanted: Caregiver for Elderly Woman; Only Family Members Need Apply*, paying family members to provide care may be an option worth considering. *"As more families face the need to care for aged parents and grandparents, some are considering a solution that might once have been shocking: paying a family member to provide care. ...It can be a great idea, as long as there are safeguards in place."* [19]

The article suggested that paying a family member can be a cost-effective alternative to getting high-quality care. Also, with the financial pressures of paying for everything from the mortgage to the day to day living expenses, few people would be able to afford quitting their jobs and then provide care for free. *"If that's what you need to do for the care of your loved one, then there should be some compensation for it."* [20]

If your family should wish to pursue this paid caregiving option, establish safeguards and agree on the role, scope of duties and responsibilities. Determine ahead of time what is to be considered paid work, what expenses are to be covered or reimbursed and more. Have a written agreement that specifies a market-based pay rate, the work schedule, how vacations and or time off would be handled and more. Also, it is suggested that families have a contingency plan in place should the caregiver unable to provide care due to illness or should the loved one's care needs becoming more complex or demanding than the family member can safely handle. [21]

Another Wall Street Journal article entitled *Who Will Take Care of Mom? Check her Family Contract* indicated a number of benefits of having a contract in place. Those benefits include: minimizing family disputes by spelling out duties; recognizing a caregiver by paying him or her for support as opposed to making adjustments to a will that might provide unequal inheritance; and, reducing the size of a person's estate through the payment for caregiving services, which may help a person qualify for Medicaid. [22]

In addition to, or instead of, paid or unpaid family caregivers, professional caregiving services can be a great way to ensure loved ones are getting the support they need and deserve when family or friends are unable to provide assistance. There are many reputable businesses that provide in-home medical (e.g., nursing) care and/or specialize in providing custodial care, also known as companion and non-medical care. For example, one such organization providing non-medical care, Home Helpers (www.HomeHelpers.CC) is based in my hometown of Cincinnati with independently owned and operated offices across North America.

Many people choose care provided by professional caregivers for the individualized attention not found in many group care and senior living environments. Care receivers also find value in maintaining their day-to-day routine and responsibilities, including housekeeping, meal preparation, getting to appointments, dealing with inconveniences, minimizing loneliness and more.

While there are pros and cons of any care arrangement, numerous studies indicate older adults prefer to remain in their home. A recent study completed by Georgetown University regarding long-term care financing found that 86% of people with long-term care needs live at home or in community settings, not in long-term care communities or institutions.[23] While home is be the preferred choice, when safety becomes an issue, regular in-home care services or moving to a different living environment may be necessary.

When considering care options and insurance coverage, be sure to find out what types of care are covered. For example, the long-term care insurance policies often cover both medical and non-medical care, where as Medicare does not cover what the government refers to as *custodial care*. Medicare defines custodial care as *"Care that can be given safely and reasonably by a person who is not medically skilled, and that is given mainly to help the patient with daily living."* [24]

Top Five Reasons Why Caregiving Is Challenging

Although everyone's situation is different, the basic challenges and predominant issues usually are the same. I find that people are better able to cope and are more apt to act when they understand the issues with which they are dealing.

Findings from research that I conducted over a three-year period indicated five main reasons family caregivers often find themselves overwhelmed and unprepared. Whether you are preparing for future responsibility or are already a caregiver, I expect you will be able to relate to the findings, and that you may even respond by thinking *that makes sense* or *now I understand.*

1. INconsistent: The age at which people begin facing functional limitations can be quite *inconsistent.* Some people age gracefully and live independently into their 80s and 90s. Others face complications or illness and need assistance in their 40s or 50s. This age inconsistency makes it difficult for families to know when to get more involved in a loved one's life. Compounding this challenge are health problems that often go undiagnosed because many people have a difficult time distinguishing characteristics of normal aging from age-related disease or illness. As a result, it often takes a crisis situation to occur for family members to take a more active role.

2. INdependent: Family caregivers and care recipients often do not seek outside support because the issues they face tend to be personal and private. Family caregivers also find it difficult to identify, and consequently associate with, others facing similar challenges. Instead, many try to figure everything out on their own. At a time when information and support is so important, the tendency is for family members to try to cope *independently* instead of reaching out for help and direction.

3. INexperienced: It does not matter what you have done as an adult or parent – nothing will prepare you to deal with age-related health concerns and long-term care. Caregivers and care recipients quickly find they are *inexperienced,* and they lack knowledge and understanding about the many issues and challenges they are likely to encounter.

Likewise, they soon realize the U.S. health care system is fragmented, specialized and difficult to navigate. For example, until people approach the age of 65, most have never given much consideration to anticipating frailty and old age, receiving care, or navigating the Social Security and Medicare system, let alone coping with dying and death.

4. INtrusive: A common response to a family member who expresses concern or a wish to provide support is "I'm fine." When that occurs, family members find themselves unsure of how to respond, how to help and what to do. Periods of change and adjustment can be extremely hard, especially on people who are aging or ill. Role conflict can be emotionally challenging. People do not want to be a burden and often find it difficult to accept support. Involvement in other people's personal affairs feels uncomfortable and *intrusive*. In addition, family members struggle with the principles of honor, obey and respect.

5. INterlocking: Although it may be human nature to focus strictly on what people perceive to be the immediate issue or problem, I find that by doing so people often get blindsided by seemingly unrelated issues. Caregiving is a process of dealing with the unexpected. Failure to look beyond the immediate issue and see the bigger picture often leads to regrets. I find that when caregivers consider the bigger picture (see diagram on next page), the *interlocking* issues, and how the choices made today affect tomorrow, they are better able to make informed decisions.

The Puzzle Pieces

Understanding the many issues associated with each puzzle piece and how they work together can help families anticipate, understand and address the challenges they are likely to face as loved ones age, become ill, or otherwise become incapacitated. The four puzzle pieces are:

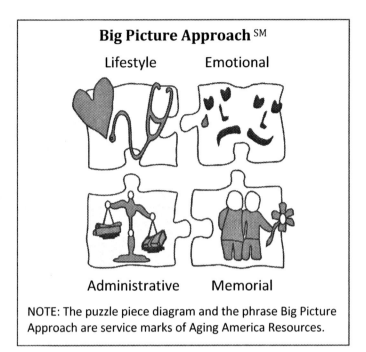

Big Picture Approach ^{SM}

Lifestyle   Emotional

Administrative   Memorial

NOTE: The puzzle piece diagram and the phrase Big Picture Approach are service marks of Aging America Resources.

- Lifestyle: This piece of the puzzle encompasses the day-to-day aspects of life, such as a person's medical condition, physical and mental functioning level, living environments, care needs, transportation, socialization and nutrition.

- Administrative: This puzzle piece focuses on legal and financial affairs, advance directives, estate planning, Social Security, Medicare, Medicaid, life insurance, long-term care insurance, scams and having *The Talk*.

- Memorial: This piece of the puzzle includes not only end-of-life issues and considerations, but also ways people can make the most of each day and preserve memories.

- Emotional: This puzzle piece covers the many heart and soul issues that people often overlook, such as understanding the care recipient's perspective, coping, managing feelings, being a confident decision-maker and identifying and engaging support resources.

The Big Picture Approach

I created the puzzle pieces diagram in 2002 having concluded from my research that, all too often, people serving the role of caregiver approach caregiving as a series of unique events or tasks instead of a process. Although it may be human nature to focus strictly on the issue at hand, failure to consider the implications of actions or inactions often leads to regrets. I find people are better able to cope and more likely to act when they see how everything fits into the big picture. They understand the many issues with which they are dealing.

Here's why this model is so important: I concluded that if a person faces an issue involving any one puzzle piece, at least two other puzzle pieces are affected. The following example should help you understand the concept. Imagine a loved one is diagnosed with an illness (a Lifestyle issue). Based on the likely trajectory of the illness, testing may be necessary and treatment decisions will need to be made. When considering the prognosis, many Lifestyle issues may need to be addressed (e.g., daily living activities, personal care, care arrangements, living environment, transportation, socialization and nutrition.)

The puzzle pieces that interlock with Lifestyle are Emotional and Administrative. Consider the Emotional issues that will likely affect the care receiver and the caregiver(s), such as accepting support, working through family dynamics, trusting in God, and dealing with feelings of anger, denial, fear and more. Also, realize that before informed medical and/or care decisions can be made, families must understand the Administrative issues. For example:

- What are your loved one's wishes and expectations?
- Has your loved one executed Advance Directives?
- Who has legal authority to make health care decisions if your loved one is unable or incapacitated?

- If necessary, who is appointed to manage his/her personal affairs?
- What does health insurance cover, and what cost may you/your loved ones be responsible for?
- Does your loved one have long-term care insurance?
- What types of financial resources are available? Are they sufficient to meet both current and future care-related expenses?

Do you see that by considering the bigger picture and understanding the issues represented by the interlocking puzzle pieces, you are more likely to make informed and thoughtful decisions?

I encourage people to avoid focusing solely on the issue at hand as doing so often leads to a false sense of security. Inexperienced caregivers often think that once they address the immediate issue, they are done. They may not realize the next challenge could be just moments or months away. As a result of not understanding how the four categories interlock, people often get blindsided by seemingly unrelated issues.

Here's another quick example of a scenario including the Memorial puzzle piece. When a loved one dies (a Memorial issue), there are associated Administrative issues (e.g. paying for a funeral, settling an estate, completing a final federal tax return) and Emotional issues (e.g. memorializing a loved one's life, mourning and grieving).

Your Turn: Can You See The Bigger Picture?

Consider a hypothetical scenario like your dad's driving, which may be a real concern. What are some of the issues or challenges you might expect to face? Think about it. Take out a sheet of paper and come up with a list of things you may want to consider. Once you have your list, compare it to my list, and see if you saw the bigger picture.

Here's the list I came up with:

- How might you determine if your dad is unsafe to drive?
- What do you do if you think dad should stop driving?
- How might you approach him to express a concern or engage him in conversation about his driving?
- What do you do if he is in denial and resists talking about driving or discussing your concerns and suggestions?
- What if he does not stop driving, and consequently injures himself, a passenger or pedestrian?
- How might you respond if he fails to pass the vision test when his license is up for renewal, and he comes home mad and upset?
- If he does stop driving, have you given consideration to how his independence and feeling of self-worth might be affected?
- How is he going to get around town if he does not drive?
- Are there alternative modes of transportation that he deems to be safe and acceptable?
- If he has to pay for transportation, are funds available?
- What will happen to the car?
- Have you thought about cancelling the insurance policy when he stops driving so he gets a refund?

Did you see the bigger picture? Many people consider an issue like driving to be something you bring up, dad agrees and you're done. The reality is that caregivers often become so distraught about what to say, how to say it and dad's response, that they never confront the issue. The point is that a single issue like driving touches upon numerous issues: Lifestyle – the choices and alternatives; Emotional – the discussion and relationship; Administrative – the financial and legal issues;

and Memorial – coping with loss. I share information and advice specific to transportation and driving in my book *Engaging While AGING*.

As I reflect on the 10 years I spent caring for my parents, I think my biggest mistake was addressing each issue or task by itself. Although it felt right at the time, with each new challenge, we were not prepared. It was mentally and physically grueling! I wish my sister and I had known to consider the pieces of the puzzle and how everything is interrelated. While it may seem obvious now, it is not what most people think about. For example, when my father was admitted into the hospital on his 79th birthday and the prognosis was not good, no one suggested we consider funeral planning until his death occurred.

Caregiving Anyone?

While caregiving should be fulfilling and rewarding for both the care receiver and caregiver(s), that does not mean it is going to be easy. Logic and good intentions often go unappreciated, and family dynamics tend to take on a whole new dimension. I offer the following perspectives to get you thinking about the emotional and practical aspects of caregiving:

1. *No one wants to care for an aging parent or ill spouse.*

   I am not suggesting people are not happy to provide needed care. Instead, I am saying we would probably all prefer that our loved ones not be in a position where care is necessary. In other words, we would prefer our loved ones to be living active and independent lifestyles as opposed to facing challenges due to aging or illness. Keep this perspective in mind when you face a tough situation. It is okay to get frustrated, just do not take it out on your loved ones.

2. *No one <u>wants</u> to become dependent on others for the essentials of daily living.*

Everyone has dreams for his or her life and retirement years. The dreams are never to become dependent on someone else for the daily essentials of basic life. Pride and stubbornness can get in the way of a loved one's willingness to accept assistance. Older adults who have been self-sufficient and independent all their lives often find it difficult to accept help. Also, people do not want to be a burden on their family. Do not be surprised if your loved ones do not graciously accept your offers and attempts to provide support. Likewise, if comments are made that upset or anger you, try not to take them personally.

3. *People do the best they <u>do not</u> know how.*

You do not do the best you know how, because if you have never dealt with issues involving aging, caregiving and long-term care, you probably have no idea what to expect and how best to help. Seeking information and direction to help you along your journey is a critical step in the caregiving process. I find that when people are aware of the issues, know their loved ones' wishes and preferences, understand the options and alternatives, and recognize the implications of their actions/inactions and decisions, they are better able to make informed decisions.

4. *People spend more time 'planning' when they should be <u>'preparing'</u>.*

Regardless of how well a person has planned for his or her retirement years, even the best laid plans can crumble. The problem with planning is that there are too many uncontrollable variables. People who plan tend to focus on the ideal situation and give very little consideration, if any, to what might be considered less than optimal scenarios. On the other hand, people who prepare tend to give thought to multiple scenarios, consider the reality that long-term care may be needed, and are better able to respond in a variety of circumstances. For example, what do you know about services available in your area such as Adult Day Stay, Senior Centers, Home Care and Assisted Living Communities. What are you waiting for? Check out some of the options and see what they are all about. What do you have to lose?

A Closing Thought

I wholeheartedly believe that caregiving should be fulfilling and rewarding for both the caregivers and care receivers. Caregiving may not be easy, but it should be rewarding. Often the difference between frustration and satisfaction is having knowledge, understanding, confidence, and courage. While caregivers often say they are overwhelmed, unprepared and uninformed, it does not have to be that way. I encourage you to apply the information and insight I share throughout this book to help you along your journey.

Life is unpredictable. As the Nationwide® Insurance television commercials (2007) say, *Life Comes At You Fast®*.[25] Whenever possible, take time to anticipate issues that you might find yourself needing to address. Making decisions in a crisis can be challenging. Emotions can confuse the issues, and options are seldom given the consideration they merit.

Be careful not to focus on the *here and now* without recognizing the many related issues. As my puzzle piece model suggests, each new issue and decision you face will impact other issues in the same puzzle piece, as well as issues in at least two other puzzle pieces.

In addition to caring for and supporting the needs and wishes of others, do not overlook planning for your own future.

I find it astonishing that most people spend more time planning for a vacation than they do preparing for the realities of aging and caregiving. I recently read an article indicating *"45% of Americans have had a personal experience caring for an aging or ill relative."* [26] It went on to say that almost half of the respondents who have had a personal caregiving experience have not taken steps to develop plans to address their own long-term care.

I encourage you to get your own affairs in order and make sure your loved ones know your wishes and expectations. Also, if you have children, keep in mind that the compassion and care you provide to your loved ones will have a lasting effect on how your children perceive how you should be treated.

Let me close this chapter with an excerpt from a letter I received a few years ago. I hope your thoughts echo this person's thoughts:

"Many thanks for your resources and taking the time to speak with me personally. I find your information and perspectives to be quite interesting and encouraging, though a bit daunting to realize all the decision points ahead."

KEY LEARNINGS – *Top three findings from this chapter:*
1.
2.
3.

ACTION ITEMS - *Things you want to do or do differently:*

Check when Completed	*Action Item*	*Target Completion Date*

"Without a sense of caring, there can be no sense of community."
– Anthony J. D'Angelo

2.

Discovering Roles and Responsibilities

Caregiving is about providing support and encouragement to help make life easier and more enjoyable for people who find aspects of daily life challenging or unsatisfying. While we hope our loved ones live long, healthy, and prosperous lives, the reality is many people require care at some point in their lives. Regardless of whether loved ones are elderly, recovering from illnesses or injuries, or otherwise need assistance, the challenges are often the same.

Quite often, adult children have limited involvement in the lives of their loved ones until a crisis occurs. It is then that they suddenly drop everything, come to the aid and begin taking a more active role. This scenario is played out in a movie I highly recommend, *DAD* (1989), and it stars Jack Lemmon, Ted Danson and Olympia Dukakis.[27] It is a wonderful portrayal of how family members rally and make life changes once the father's care needs are recognized.

Is It Time To Get More Involved?

One question I am regularly asked is, *"How do I know if my loved one needs or could benefit from assistance?"* To answer this question, I wrote an article in the fall of 2002 entitled *Holiday 'Check-Ups' – Are My Aging Parents Okay?* The article begins:

> *"Over the River and Through the Woods ..." As families gather for the holidays, many might overlook their aging parents' behavior, thinking that it is a senior moment or normal aging, when in fact, there may be a reason for concern. Charles Puchta offers a few holiday tips for families with aging or ill loved ones.*
>
> *"Holiday visits are a wonderful time to informally "check-up" on older family members, as gatherings are usually longer than the more typical short stop-by visits," says Puchta.*
>
> *Longer visits provide an opportunity to observe older people in a variety of situations. Many older people struggle unnecessarily and try to hide problems from the rest of the family because they do not want to impose upon them or worry them."*

On Nov. 17, 2002, The Wall Street Journal featured a story based on my article entitled *Are Mom and Dad OK?* An excerpt of the story is as follows:

> *" ... here's some help to figure out whether your folks are all right on their own. Author and aging expert Charles Puchta ... has developed a quiz to help adult children play detective, so they can figure out if it's time to offer their parents some help ... "* [28]

The article went on to share 10 questions to help family members assess functional abilities and determine if a loved one(s) may be at risk or need assistance. It is important to realize that an aging parent or ill spouse may not proactively ask for help. Many older people place a high value on their privacy and have been self-sufficient most of their lives. Others may not wish to recognize and acknowledge their struggles, or they simply do not want to be a burden. Often it is up to the adult children to recognize a parent's limitations and offer assistance and encouragement.

An assessment also is important because caregivers are *often too close to the forest to see the trees.* In other words, we may not recognize limitations that gradually increase over time. Think about it. If you do not see loved ones for an extended period of time, changes are more obvious than when you see them daily. Regardless of how often you see your loved ones, most people do not know the competencies they should regularly assess to determine if it is time to get more involved in their loved ones' lives. Review the following *10 [questions] Considerations* to help you determine if it might be time to get more involved and help a loved one address challenges he or she may be facing.

10 Considerations

1. Medical Condition – Has your loved one been diagnosed with a disease, illness or other medical condition that could impact his or her ability to function in daily life?

2. Driving – If your loved one drives, is there reason to believe he or she poses an above-average risk for being involved in an accident? How is your loved one's vision, reflexes and ability to respond in an unexpected situation?

3. Food/Nutrition – Is your loved one eating balanced meals? Is his or her weight stable? Does he or she have a reasonable variety of food in the refrigerator with future expiration dates?

4. Hygiene – Does it appear your loved one is bathing and brushing his or her teeth regularly? How is his or her

overall appearance, grooming and ability to match clothing compared to prior years? Are the bed linens and towels fresh? Does the soap in the bathroom appear have been used recently?

5. Behavior – Does your loved one seem anxious or irritable? Does being away from home make him or her uncomfortable? Does he or she seem depressed? Is there inconsistency in the things he or she says? Does your loved one remember names, places and current events?

6. Daily Tasks – Are basic tasks, such as getting ready to go out, preparing a meal or shopping, overly challenging, frustrating or time-consuming for your loved one? Does the living space appear clean? Is there concern about hoarding?

7. Medication – Can your loved one manage his or her medications properly including dosage, frequency and changes to prescriptions? Does your loved one understand why he or she is taking the medications? Are prescriptions getting refilled in a timely fashion?

8. Finances – Does it appear that your loved one is capable of making sound financial decisions? Is he or she able to manage personal affairs and finances? Does he or she have a reasonable amount of cash on hand? Have there been any unusual purchases or suspicious expenses or investments?

9. Mail – Is the mail stacking up? Is there reason to suspect any past due or delinquency notices? Does your loved one appear to be a target for solicitation and sweepstakes offers?

10. Safety – Is your loved one careful about turning off appliances (e.g. stove, coffee pot)? Does he or she ever carelessly leave candles or cigarettes burning? Are sharp objects properly put away? Are the stairs and hallways unobstructed? Are the doors and windows locked? Is he or

she able to easily locate the keys? Is there any reason to believe someone is trying to control or take advantage of him or her?

Whenever possible, I suggest you try to observe loved ones in a variety of situations. Ideally, evaluations should be informal so as not to cause alarm or appear disrespectful. Trust your instincts. If you have any concerns, even with one issue, it may be time to take a more active role in a loved one's life. Chances are that your loved one may be struggling unnecessarily, and it could be time to explore ways to help in a proactive fashion, rather than waiting to react. Depending on the severity of your concerns, you may also want to seek professional advice from you loved one's health care providers (e.g., doctor, home care agency, hospice provider), an Area Agency on Aging or a national organization such as the Alzheimer's Association. If you wish to speak with any of your parent's medical providers, a HIPPA release may be required before they can share information or discuss your loved one's medical condition with you.

NOTE: If your concerns lead you to believe that there may be imminent danger, speak with a health care professional immediately to determine what type of treatment or support may be necessary. You might also visit www.ElderCareLocator.org or contact your local Area Agency on Aging (AAA). For a complete listing of AAAs visit: www.n4a.org/answers-on-aging.

Should you identify one or more areas of concern, talk to your loved one in a casual and non-threatening way. Ideally, your conversations should reflect a partnership and demonstrate a desire and willingness to respect your loved one's wishes and address his or her struggles. I suggest you and your family begin by acknowledging any concern(s) and determine if other family members have similar concerns. In addition, to help defuse potential conflicts and possible fears, I highly recommend you assure your loved one(s) that your intent is to understand and respect his or her wishes while providing support and care.

Often there are simple things caregivers can do to provide assistance. I encourage you to be proactive. What may begin as kind gestures can help the care receiver value the support and build trust. In the following chapters, I elaborate on ways you can address potential areas of concern. For example:

- Medical Condition – Go with your parent or loved one to his/her next doctor's appointment and listen to what the doctor has to say. It is not uncommon for an older person to avoid asking questions as he or she might not want to hear what the doctor has to say or may not be able to process and understand what is being said.

- Driving – If your parent drives, let him or her drive when you go out to lunch or run an errand. Observe your loved one's driving skills and determine if his or her abilities present concerns. If you have concern, learn about the programs and alternatives that might be appropriate.

- Food/Nutrition – Offer to help with grocery shopping, make an extra casserole each week for a loved one, or look into organizations and programs that deliver meals.

- Hygiene – If towels, linens or clothes do not appear fresh, offer to do an occasional load of laundry or suggest outside assistance. Tasks that may be easy for a younger person may be more challenging to others. Do not assume. Ask how you can help.

- Behavior – If a person is showing unusual behavior, try to determine if there are certain times of the day or situations where the behaviors are more extreme. If there are situations that cause anxiety such as crowds and noise (e.g., over-stimulation), try to avoid them. Provide reassurance to the person that *"It's going to be okay"* and seek medical help as you deem appropriate.

- Daily Tasks – Determine if there are daily tasks you can perform to help lighten the load. Give consideration to the ability and comfort level of others to perform certain tasks, particularly when a spouse suddenly finds him or herself alone.

- Medications – See if there are ways to help with medications, such as sorting pills into day-of-the-week dispensers. Also, consider placing reminders in the house or making a reminder phone call. Keep a list of all medications including dosage, frequency, purpose, prescribing medical professional and expected refill date.

- Finances – Keeping up-to-date on finances can be difficult for some people. With advances like online banking and automatic bill payment services, it is easier for a family member to provide assistance.

- Mail – As people age, their behavior regarding mail often changes. What was once considered junk mail is often opened and kept. I suggest family members warn loved ones about scams and tactics to get people to buy things they do not need. Encourage your loved one to be aware and get a second opinion before buying.

- Safety – Walk around your loved one's home and see if there is anything that concerns you – overloaded extension cords, wobbly furniture or railings, area rugs that could be trip hazards. Take steps to ensure your loved one's home is as safe as possible.

While caregiving often involves daily tasks, I believe it is important for you as a caregiver to keep in mind that you are supporting a person who matters and has feelings. All too often, I find that caregivers become so focused on the tasks and trying to *fix things* that they overlook their loved one's need for relationship, companionship, and social engagement.

Geriatric Functional Assessment

If, as a result of your informal assessment, you have safety concerns or believe that a loved one is not functioning at an age-appropriate level, a formal assessment may be appropriate. A Geriatric Assessment or Functional Assessment provides an opportunity to seek expert input on a person's physical, mental and psychological functioning.

Why Conduct A Functional Assessment?

1. Family members are often too close to a situation to be objective. As a result, many people simply do not see impairments, limitations, potential hazards and other challenges. Loved ones may also hide or cover up things. *My parents proved to be experts at masking things. By the time my sister and I realized my mom's limitations, we were shocked to find she was functioning at a much lower level than we ever imagined.*

2. Many people simply do not know or do not want to admit to themselves that their capabilities have diminished over the years. For example, I know many people in their 40s and 50s that already are having difficulty driving at night. The point is that if younger baby boomers are already experiencing vision changes that make their driving abilities unsafe in certain conditions, and they still drive, imagine the challenges older people may be facing but are not willing to acknowledge or admit.

3. Older people often find everyday activities to be more complex and difficult than in their younger years. A task or activity in and of itself may be easy. But when they try to combine five or six tasks, they may become overwhelmed and find it difficult to cope.

4. Just as *too many cooks spoil the broth"* counsel from too many people can cause conflict. Take, for example, a situation where an older person is seeing several doctors for many conditions. Occasionally, the doctors will prescribe medications for different conditions without knowledge of other medications the person taking subjecting the person to possible adverse side effects.

5. A Functional Assessment identifies challenges a loved one may be encountering with basic bodily functions and issues affecting one's dignity. As adults age, they may need assistance with bathing, toileting, grooming, dressing and more.

The Functional Assessment is a wonderful tool to provide loved ones and family members with reliable and accurate information needed to assess a situation and begin to make informed decisions. An Assessment is often a series of studies conducted by a variety of health care professionals (e.g., doctor, nurse, physical/occupational therapist, social worker), using a variety of formats, including one-on-one conversations and interactive exercises. The Assessment can help to identify areas in which a person is functioning below the norm. It also pinpoints challenges and limitations that may hinder a person's ability to independently care for him or herself and function in everyday society.

To discuss the benefits of a Comprehensive Geriatric Assessments and see if one might be appropriate for your loved one, you might speak with your parent's doctor. As mentioned earlier in the chapter, before a medical doctor is able to share information, a HIPPA release signed by your loved one that grants you permission to know personal medical information is necessary. To identify medical practices that conduct Geriatric Assessments you might contact the local Area on Agency or visit: www.americangeriatrics.org. The specifics of an assessment may vary by state, medical facility and doctor. A health care professional can help you determine the most appropriate solution and explain the assessment alternatives available in your community. Keep in mind that with the combination of a decreasing number of medical professionals in the field of Geriatric Medicine, and more people seeking a Functional Assessment, it can often be months before someone can be seen by a geriatric specialist for an assessment.

Components of a Comprehensive Geriatric Assessment include:

- Review of concerns and what family members are hoping to accomplish.
- Review of patient information, medical and family history.
- Review of medications being taken and why.
- Comprehensive medical exam, including review of bodily systems and mental health.
- Review of nutritional and sleep patterns.

Because many conditions affecting the elderly are common and expected, a Geriatric Assessment is a great way to determine if there is reason for concern. You can work with medical professionals and social workers to tailor solutions based on individual needs, to either improve or maintain your loved one's functional abilities and quality of life. Common issues center on a person's mobility, grooming and personal care. Other issues may include ensuring adequate nutrition, money management, societal and environment issues and a loved one's ability to safely operate and control a motor vehicle.

What Does Caregiving Entail?

I find many people underestimate what is involved in providing compassionate care. When you think of caregiving, what comes to mind? I find most people think about the more tangible aspects of caregiving because that is what is more often written about.

For example, according to the Pfizer Journal entitled *A Profile of Caregiving in America (2005)*, over 80% of caregivers provide assistance with daily living activities, such as providing transportation, grocery shopping and other essentials, housekeeping, managing finances, preparing meals, dispensing medications and more.[29] In addition to performing *tasks*, caregivers also serve in many different *roles*. Some of the more common roles include:

- Advisor – Offering recommendations to help a loved one identify potential challenges, talking about concerns, sharing information and considering alternatives that may help to maximize his or her independence and quality of life.

- Advocate – Looking out for a loved one's best interests as an authorized agent (e.g., Power of Attorney). Ensuring the person you serve gets the information, care, support and treatment he or she needs and deserves.

- Coordinator – Arranging for services, such as professional caregiving, physical therapy, lawn mowing, snow removal and heating/air conditioning repair, scheduling appointments, coordinating deliveries, helping to facilitate end-of-life planning and more.

- Evaluator – Assessing a loved one's ability to live independently, handle his or her own personal care, manage medications, operate a motor vehicle and more. Also, identifying and evaluating appropriate programs and services that best match a care receiver's needs and wishes.

- Mediator – Helping family members and others communicate with health care and social service providers, make decisions and resolve issues in a positive and helpful manner.

- Protector – Taking charge when necessary to help ensure the safety and wellbeing of a loved one.

- Provider – Providing assistance when a loved one is not able to care for him or herself due to physical or cognitive limitations. Assistance often addresses the following types of needs:

  o Emotional – Listening and responding to concerns, providing encouragement and moral support, and simply being there for someone.

  o Financial – Organizing bills, writing checks, balancing the checkbook, and providing money to help cover expenses.

  o Physical – Assisting with daily living activities, including personal care, household chores, meals, driving, etc.

  o Social – Maintaining regular contact and minimizing isolation and boredom through relationship and keeping loved ones "in the loop".

  o Spiritual – Helping people find meaning and purpose in life, maintaining hope, coping and finding peace through prayer, meditation and cultural and religious preferences.

Often, the demands of caregiving have an adverse effect on a caregiver's work, wallet and way of life. According to a John Hancock survey (2006), many Americans are impacted by caregiving for aging family members and friends: *"Nearly 7 in 10 (69%) respondents said that providing care and/or assistance significantly affected their personal lives, and 62% said that it had a significant impact on family. Almost half (45%) said that caregiving significantly affected their work ... Of those who provide financial assistance, over one third (36%) pay more than $1,000 per month..."* [30]

A 2007 study conducted by the National Alliance for Caregiving and Evercare found that the average annual out-of-pocket expense associated with caregiving for the elderly is approximately $5,500 when both the caregiver(s) and care receiver are local, and a little more than $8,700 when the caregiver(s) is out of town or *long-distance*.[31] The study is significant in that the cost figures are considerably higher than previous estimates and more than the annual entertainment and health care expenses combined for the average household in America.

Long-Distance Caregiving

While the roles and responsibilities are vast, being long distance can often involve a monkey wrench or two thrown into the equation. For example, what if you live in a different city, state or country? In today's culture, it is common for family to live apart from one another. A son or daughter may move to a distant city for a job or marriage. Parents may seek a change in lifestyle or climate upon retirement. Just because you live out-of-town does not mean you cannot be a caregiver. Instead, you are considered a *long-distance caregiver*.

According to the National Institute on Aging, approximately 15% of all caregivers, or seven million adults, are long-distance caregivers.[32] Long-distance caregivers are people who provide support for a loved one living an hour or more away. People who regularly travel for business, even though they may live in the same city, face many of the same challenges as long-distance caregivers. While the type of support a person provides tends to be different when he or she is out-of-town, there are many ways to be supportive regardless of distance.

Being out-of-town is challenging and may be considered a disadvantage as it can be difficult to know how loved ones are functioning and coping with everyday activities. I share two recommendations for long-distance caregivers:

1. Engage Professional – Often there are professionals, such as in-home caregivers and/or a geriatric care manager that can work with you to manage or oversee the care. In addition, professionals can provide updates so you can stay informed about a loved one's health and wellbeing.

2. Notify Your Employer – Should you suddenly need to leave town or make personal phone calls during work hours to coordinate care or speak with a health care professional, it can be helpful if your boss is in the know. Also, if you notify your employer of your role as a long-distance caregiver, you might contact your company's human resources department to ask about elder care benefits (e.g., back-up elder care, referral services, long-term care insurance, Family Medical Leave) which you may not be aware. For information about the Family Medical Leave Act visit: www.dol.gov/esa/whd/fmla.

For more information about long-distance caregiving, you might request a free resource entitled *So Far Aware, Twenty Questions for Long-Distance Caregivers* from the National Institute on Aging – www.nia.nih.gov or (301) 496-1752. Also, visit the Family Caregiver Alliance website at Caregiver.org and search for the *Handbook for Long-Distance Caregivers*.

Family Dynamics

In addition to distance, family dynamics can also present some challenges. Although most people have good intentions, the care process can be challenging and good intentions are not always recognized. Likewise, past hurts and rivalries often emerge (e.g., Miss Goody Two Shoes, *"Mom always liked you better."*) While it may not be easy to do, I suggest family members put the past behind them and focus on the future for the benefit of loved ones in need. Also, if stepparents or stepchildren are involved, it can complicate matters and introduce many other issues that may need to be considered and addressed.

Differences of opinion, understanding and style often become apparent as family members participate in the care process. While this may present some unexpected or unwelcome frustrations, know that people and their approaches are different. I tend to be the thinker – I want to take charge and fix things. On the other hand, my wife is more of a feeler and believes her presence, the relationship, is more important than taking action. Whether you are more focused on *doing* or *being*, one is not good or bad, right or wrong – they are just different.

I hope the following example will help you recognize that we all do things differently each and every day. Think of a situation ... buying a sweater, selecting a new car, or ordering off of a menu. The commonality is that, in each of these situations, you have choices. And, as you know, people often do not come to the same conclusions. For example, I would never buy a black car because I have always believed that dark-colored cars show the dirt too easily. However, that does not mean the millions of people who drive black cars are foolish. The point I am trying to make is that we will always have differences of opinion. Often, our differences can be our strengths and can help families come together and share responsibilities for a common purpose – caregiving.

So the question is, when multiple people are involved in the care process, are each person's contributions valued equally? One of the things I always tell my kids when they make the comment *"That's not fair"* is, *"You're right. It's not fair, and frankly, you would not want fair."* The goal is to try and make things as equitable as possible, but that may be quite different in terms of roles and responsibilities.

Another matter to consider is that everyone has different availabilities and methods of coping. Some siblings and other family members (e.g., in-laws) may not be able to provide assistance during normal working hours. Others may have prior commitments or obligations during the evenings or weekends. In terms of coping methods, some people accept and address issues head on, while others take a more passive approach or are in denial. As I am sure you already know, people respond to situations differently. We cannot force people to do things our way. Instead, I suggest:

- Being Sensitive to One Another – We all have people who rely on us in one way or another. However, many family caregivers, both local and long-distance, may feel they are either providing the majority of support or not doing enough. Make sure to recognize each other's contributions, provide encouragement and show your appreciation.

- Defining Roles – If two or more family members can provide support, it is helpful to share the responsibilities. Begin by considering each other's strengths and limitations. Determine what needs to be handled locally and what can be done from out-of-town. For example, coordinating services, scheduling appointments, advising loved ones of options, handling insurance claims, paying bills and more can often be handled at different times of the day or night and can even be handled remotely. Also, while providing a hand to help meet someone's physical needs may not be possible, helping to meet a loved one's emotional, financial and spiritual needs may be.

Regardless of family dynamics, where you live or your availability to help with the more routine or daily aspects of caregiving, I suggest all family members give consideration to the following:

- Know What to Expect – Learn as much as you can about your loved ones' medical concerns, including symptoms, diagnosis, treatment and self-management of an illness or disease. Consider how their daily living or functioning may be affected and what type of assistance they may need, both now and in the future. Rather than waiting for a crisis to occur, try to anticipate needs and plan ahead.

- Be Prepared – Maintain and keep handy a contact list of friends and neighbors – both yours and your parents – in case of an emergency. Friends and neighbors may also be helpful should you have a concern and need someone to visit your parents and make sure they are okay. Have a game plan just in case you need to get home quickly. Keep a Yellow Pages phone book (hard copy or online version) nearby should you need assistance from an organization in your parent's hometown.

- Maintain Regular Contact – Be supportive of your parents and your siblings. Simple actions can go a long way, such as asking how you can help or calling daily. Offering words of encouragement and support to siblings who are taking a more active role is often much appreciated. For long-distance caregivers and others who are unable to make regular visits, hearing a loved one's voice over the phone can help bridge the distance. When you talk with one another, ask specific and open-ended questions to get a sense of how your parents/siblings are truly doing. For example, *"Has mom been taking her medication on schedule?" "What was the highlight of your day?" Or, "What was the most difficult or frustrating part of our day?"*

- Plan Your Visits – Chances are your loved ones are eagerly awaiting your next visit. Longer visits provide an opportunity to observe people in a variety of situations. Informally assess your parents' health, wellbeing and safety. Many older adults, and those who are ill, struggle unnecessarily and try to hide problems from the rest of the family because they do not want to impose upon them or worry them. Whenever possible, try to coordinate visits at a time your parents may have check-ups or appointments so you can go with them.

- Seek Outside Support – In addition to seeking services to help make day-to-day life easier, you may consider hiring someone to be your eyes and ears and help keep you regularly informed, such as a geriatric care manager (GCM). To locate the names of GCMs in your area visit the website o the National Association of Professional Geriatric Care Managers at: www.CareManger.org. Also, attending a caregiver support group can help you manage your feelings and gain perspectives from others. Your local Area Agency on Aging can direct you to local support groups.

- Use Technology – For peace of mind, encourage your parents to use a GPS system if they drive and keep a cell phone with when away from their home. Some newer cell phones designate emergency contacts with red lettering. If a cell phone is older and does not have emergency numbers I suggest you preprogram two or three *ICE* numbers referring to *I*n *C*ase of *E*mergency (e.g., ICE #1 Robert – (987) 555-1234). Other safety solutions you may wish to explore include:

  o Comfort Zone™ – A service of the Alzheimer's Association, Comfort Zone is a location management system designed for people with dementia that enables tracking of a loved one's whereabouts using a web-based application that sends alert notification when a loved one goes outside of his or her designated safe zone.

  o PERS – A personal emergency response system (e.g., "I've fallen and need help") can be an important part of an overall care program, enabling a system user to get assistance when in a predicament or help in the case of an emergency. With the press of a button on the pendent or base unit, the monitoring service will initiate a response.

o   Safe Return® – A service of MedicAlert® + Alzheimer's Association, Safe Return® is a 24-hour nationwide emergency response service for individuals with dementia who wander or have a medical emergency. The medic alert bracelet provides key information to help emergency personal respond appropriately.

Developing A Care Plan

While understanding the various facets of caregiving is important, a challenge for many people is putting their knowledge into practice. Developing a care plan can be a helpful way to address known needs and put good intentions into action. A care plan essentially addresses *What, Who* and *How.*

Questions to consider include:

- What specific care or assistance is needed and anticipated?

- Who in the family will share the caregiving responsibility?

- How will the responsibilities be shared (e.g., designated tasks and responsibilities for each person)?

- Who will take on the primary family caregiver role?

- What is the availability of family members to serve as caregivers?

- What skills or training might be needed by caregivers to perform functions properly and safely?

My sister and I divided the responsibilities for the care of our parents. I took the lead for our dad, and she took the lead for our mom. This way, we were better able to address any male/female concerns. My sister also handled scheduling medical appointments and made most healthcare decisions. I took the lead handling personal and administrative matters.

Give some thought to the responsibilities for your situation and who may be able to provide needed assistance. If you have a sibling(s) and find yourself in a situation where it seems like you are doing all the work, and few or none of the responsibilities are being shared, ask for help. When one family member is serving as a primary caregiver, he or she can often become exhausted and resentful that others are not doing more to help. Quite often, siblings have no idea how much time and effort someone is spending providing care and support. I often tell caregivers not to get mad at their sibling(s) for not helping more. Instead, take it as a compliment that you are doing such a good job – maybe too good.

If you feel as though the weight of the world is on your shoulders and everyone else is going about their day, I suggest you keep a detailed list of all the things you are doing on a daily basis and how much time is involved. It is often not until family members become aware of the demands of caregiving that they do more to help. If this is the case with your family, I encourage you to share your list with your family so they can better understand all that is involved. Also, take the opportunity to indicate things that you need help with, point out responsibilities that do not require your physical presence, and ask for help.

In situations where your family is unable to provide the needed level of care, make sure you understand the care options that might be available in your area, and decide which option(s) is best for your situation. Regardless of whether care is provided by a family member, friend or care professional, it is important to keep in mind the following three "*P's*":

- Purpose: A natural reaction of caregivers is to over-care for a loved one. A good slogan to keep in mind is *"Help only when help is necessary."* I suggest caregivers resist the urge to complete tasks on a loved one's behalf unless assistance is requested or necessary. Just because you might be able to complete a task more quickly or easily does not mean you should do it. In fact, many care receivers indicate it is demoralizing with others take over and do the things they are capable of doing themselves.

- Provide: Encourage the use of assistive devices and make arrangements as appropriate that enable a loved one to maintain his or her mobility (e.g., a cane, walker or wheelchair) and independence (e.g., use of hearing and vision aids, dentures and other adaptive devices.)

- Preserve: Always provide care in a manner that preserves a person's dignity, offers choices and encourages participation. Remember that the loss of ability and dependence upon others is often frustrating, humiliating and discouraging.

If your care plan involves providing physical assistance, be sure you know how to do so safely. There are specific techniques for helping people transfer from a bed to a chair, helping a person up from the toilet, assisting someone in and out of a bathtub or in and out of a car. To learn the various techniques and prevent injury to yourself, seek training and assistance.

NOTE: When providing personal care, it is important to do so safely and in a way that provides dignity and privacy. To learn techniques for assisting with bathing, grooming, mouth care, dressing, toileting and more, I recommend an America Red Cross (ARC) publication entitled *Assisting with Personal Care* Stock No. 653985. To obtain a copy, contact your local chapter or call the ARC National Headquarters at (202) 303-5000.

Red Flag Reactions

There are several natural reactions that are common to people taking on the role of family caregiver. I share these scenarios to help you understand the care recipient's viewpoint.

Reaction #1: *"What Am I Going To Do?"*

When a loved one faces a crisis situation, it is common for a family caregiver's response to be *"What am I going to do?"* I suggest that before *you* do anything, you put yourself in the shoes of the care recipient. Gerontology classes at universities across the country often conduct exercises to help students better appreciate the realities many older adults face. From putting tape over your glasses so you cannot see as clearly, and putting cotton in your ears to muffle sound, to restricting your legs so you are forced to shuffle, you will quickly come to appreciate the limitations loved ones may face.

Reaction #2: *Treat People Differently*

When a loved one faces a challenge or is labeled with a medical condition, family and friends have a tendency to treat the person differently. I suggest that you treat the person the same as before a medical condition existed. Instead, what you should treat differently is the circumstances. Let me say that again. *Do not treat the person differently, treat the circumstances differently.* When I talk about the circumstances, I am focusing on the environment as opposed to the person. For example, say a person is experiencing hearing loss. Treat the person with the same loving kindness as before. To address the circumstance of hearing loss, you might reduce background noises, speak slower and louder, and enunciate your words more clearly. If a person has dementia, it is important to treat the circumstances differently to help reduce potential anxiety, agitation or confusion. Do not put your loved one on the spot by asking a complex question or over-stimulating them.

Reaction #3: *"Let Me Do That"*

Regardless of whether a person's limitation is a result of age, illness or injury, a natural tendency for family and friends is to overcompensate for them. I call this the *"Let Me"* mentality. Although your gestures may seem like the right thing to do, they are often unnecessary and even demoralizing. One question I frequently receive is: *"Why do you think so many older people resist assistance from family members?"* Many people think the answer is that older people are stubborn or set in their ways. I have a different philosophy. My guess is that people are hesitant to place themselves in a situation where they become vulnerable. For example, if a loved one accepts a family member's assistance with one activity, how is he or she going to say no the next time a son or daughter offers to help? They decline help instead of having someone come in, take over and start doing things a different way.

The movie *Driving Miss Daisy* clearly portrays the *"Let Me"* concept. Without input or interest from the mother, played by Jessica Tandy, the son, played by Dan Ackroyd, hires Morgan Freeman as his mother's chauffeur. Ackroyd also tells Freeman that he works for him, not his mother, and that she cannot fire him. When Ackroyd shows up at his mother's house to introduce her to Freeman, she is not happy about the idea of a stranger in her house eating her food and breaking her china. She also makes the comment, *"Last I knew, I had rights ..."* suggesting it was not Ackroyd's business or responsibility to take over.[33]

Caregiver Concerns

People taking on the caregiver role often find themselves in unexpected and unfamiliar situations. Also, there is a tendency for the caregivers' health to suffer as they provide care for a loved one. The Alzheimer's Association suggests being mindful of the following *10 Warning Signs of Caregiver Stress*: [34]

1. Denial about the disease and its effects on the person who has been diagnosed – *"I know mom is going to get better."*

2. Anger at the person with Alzheimer's. – *"If he asks me that question one more time, I'll scream."*

3. Social withdrawal from friends and activities – *"I do not care about getting together ... anymore."*

4. Anxiety about facing another day and what the future holds – *"What happens when he needs more care than I can provide?"*

5. Depression begins to affect the ability to cope – *"I do not care anymore."*

6. Exhaustion makes it nearly impossible to complete necessary daily tasks – *"I'm too tired for this."*

7. Sleeplessness caused by a never-ending list of concerns – *"What if she wanders out of the house or falls and hurts herself?"*

8. Irritability leads to moodiness and triggers negative responses and reactions – *"Leave me alone."*

9. Lack of concentration makes it difficult to perform familiar tasks – *"I was so busy, I forgot we had an appointment."*

10. Health problems begin to take their toll, both mentally and physically – *"I cannot remember the last time I felt good."*

In addition to being aware of your own personal stress, these warning signs may also be applicable of one parent is caring for the other. You might share this information, express your concerns, and encourage the caregiving parent to accept more assistance from adult children and/or seek the support of professional caregivers.

Some of the ways you might be able to reduce or minimize your stress include:

- Becoming educated about the illness or ailment and how it is likely to impact a person.

- Learning about caregiving and helpful techniques.
- Seeking assistance from family, friends and community resources.
- Taking care of yourself by eating right, exercising and getting plenty of rest.
- Taking some time away (a.k.a. Respite) to rejuvenate.
- Accepting changes as they occur and adapting to new situations.
- Being realistic about what you can do.
- Keeping a journal and expressing yourself on paper.
- Giving yourself credit for what you have accomplished; do not feel guilty if you lose your patience or cannot do everything on your own.

The Rights And Responsibilities Of A Caregiver

Caregiver burnout is a real concern that many people overlook. A natural tendency for many family caregivers is to unselfishly give of themselves, neglect their own care, and overdo it. A recent study by the Harvard Medical School found caregiver burnout often leads to serious illness or death of the caregiver. According to the findings, the more physically or mentally disabling a person's condition, the greater effect it will have on the health of the person serving as primary caregiver.[35]

While the study specifically made mention of spousal caregivers, burnout is a universal concern. I believe the point is that caregivers need to recognize their own limitations to maintain a healthy attitude and not feel guilty if they are not able to do everything. Burnout often takes its toll emotionally, physically, spiritually, and even financially. Finding a life balance that works for you can be tremendously valuable and help to minimize negative consequences.

Many caregivers are reluctant to ask others for support and believe they are the only ones qualified to provide care. Sometimes we need to take a step back, reach out to others and accept support. By taking care of ourselves, we are better able to help ensure our loved ones receive the care and support they need and deserve. To assess how caregiving may be affecting you, review *The Modified Caregiver Strain Index,* available at www.nursingcenter.com/pdf.asp?AID=812527. It is a tool with 13-questions that can help you screen for strain as a long-term family caregiver.

People providing care and support for a family member may find the Caregiver Bill of Rights to be helpful. The document is believed to have first been published by the AARP, and it is designed to help caregivers recognize their responsibilities and limitations.

There are many versions of The Caregiver's Bill of Rights. The one that follows is attributed to the Cincinnati Catholic Charities Southwest Ohio Caregiver Assistance Network:

1. "I have the right to take care of myself. This is not an act of selfishness. It will give me the capability of taking better care of my care receiver.
2. I have the right to occasionally get angry, be depressed, and express other difficult feelings.
3. I have the right to reject attempts by my care receiver (either conscious or unconscious) to manipulate me through guilt and/or depression.
4. I have the right to take pride in what I am doing and to applaud the courage it sometimes takes to meet the needs of the person I am caring for.
5. I have the right to appreciation and emotional support for my decision to accept the challenge of providing care.
6. I have the right to protect my assets and financial future without severing my relationship with the care receiver.

7. I have the right to respite care during emergencies and to care for my own health, spirit and relationships.

8. I have the right to provide care at home as long as it is physically, financially and emotionally feasible; however, when it is no longer feasible, I am obligated to explore other alternatives, such as a residential care community.

9. I have the right to maintain facets of my own life that do not include the person I care for, just as I would if he or she were healthy. I know that I do everything that I reasonably can for this person, and I have the right to do some things just for myself.

10. I have the right to protect my individuality and make a life for myself that will sustain me when my care receiver no longer needs my help.

11. I have the right to seek help from others even though my care receiver may object. I recognize the limits of my own endurance and strength.

12. I have the right to expect all family members, men and women, to participate in the care of aging relatives.

13. I have the right to receive consideration, affection, forgiveness and acceptance for what I do for my loved one for as long as I offer these qualities in return.

14. I have the right to temporarily change my living environment as needed to aid in caring for aging care recipients.

15. I have the right to expect professionals, in their area of specialization, to recognize the importance of palliative care and to be knowledgeable about the concerns and options related to older people and caregivers.

16. I have the right to sensitive, supportive responses by employers in dealing with unexpected or severe care needs.

17. I have the right to receive training in caregiving skills, along with accurate understandable information about the condition and needs of the care recipient.

18. I have the right to expect and demand that as new strides are made in finding resources to aid physically and mentally impaired persons in our country, similar strides will be made toward aiding and supporting caregivers." [36]

A Closing Thought

When a loved one is diagnosed with a medical condition, hospitalized or facing challenges, family members and friends are often the ones to drop everything and come to one's aid. While it seems that everyone has jam-packed schedules, it is amazing how health-related issues can instantaneously get people to reprioritize everything.

When taking on the role of caregiver, you will quickly find yourself dealing with issues you never expected. Caregiving can be difficult. Moreover, many family members do not view themselves as a *caregiver*. Determining when a person crosses the line between being a concerned, loving family member to family caregiver can be challenging. This is especially true for people who start off doing an occasional task and find their responsibility grows over time.

I believe that it is important for you to recognize yourself as a caregiver for one primary reason. Once someone declares that they are a caregiver, I find that the person is more likely to seek information, such as this book, and reach out to individuals and community-based organizations for support and direction.

A recent article in The Wall Street Journal entitled *Heartbreaking Work* so eloquently stated: *"Caregiver is a deceptively professional sounding term for a role in which most of us are complete amateurs, and for one that is apt to descend upon us like a blow from fate, stunning and unforeseen."* [37] The article went on to state *"The personal sacrifice involved in caregiving becomes its own reward."* [38]

While I believe caregivers need to understand their roles, responsibilities and rights, they also need to understand the importance of relationships. As award-winning actress S. Epatha Merkerson of the television series Law & Order said, *"As a friend and caregiver, my most important job was simply to be there* [for two of her friends struggling with lung cancer] *when they needed me and provide them with a face of courage and love."* [39] Whether providing support and encouragement to family or friends, *being* a companion is often more appreciated and valued than *doing tasks*. Often our (physical) presence is the best present.

KEY LEARNINGS – *Top three findings from this chapter:*
1.
2.
3.

ACTION ITEMS - *Things you want to do or do differently:*

Check when Completed	*Action Item*	*Target Completion Date*

> *"The great thing about getting
> older is that you do not lose all
> the other ages you've been."*
> – Madeleine L'Engle

3.

Exploring the Aging Process

In 1864, poet Robert Browning captured the hope that so many of us hold about aging: *"Grow old along with me! The best is yet to be."* [40] While the aging process is gradual and natural, unfavorable stereotypes and myths often lead people to focus on the losses and overlook and under-appreciate the gifts of aging. Many older adults find a renewed sense of purpose spending time with their grandkids, socializing with friends, pursuing hobbies, traveling and more. As a retired teacher once told a colleague of mine, one of the best things about aging is, *"The older I get, the less I feel I have to prove anything to anybody."* [41]

Believing myths about aging can in fact deny older adults opportunities and potentially lead to harm. For example, people who believe the myth, *"You cannot teach an old dog new tricks,"* may not encourage older adults to learn how to self-manage an illness or may think sharing beneficial information is pointless. To those who believe this myth, my response is that the good news is we are not teaching dogs, and we are not teaching tricks.

As for the myth, *"The horse is out the barn,"* which suggests it is too late to change bad habits and risky behaviors, the truth is that healthy choices at any age can lead to a renewed sense of wellness and quality of life. Believing the myth may limit education and encouragement that can lead to improved health.

There are many different theories about the aging process. They range from postulating that a person only has so much energy to expend in a lifetime, to suggesting that a lower calorie intake will extend life, to Hayflicks limit that indicates human cells can only divide 20 times before dying.[42] Regardless of which theory(ies) is most accurate and whether genetics or lifestyle choices and environmental factors have a greater influence on the way people age, one thing is for certain: Every- one's experience with aging and growing old is unique. While there are similarities, there are so many factors that shape a person's life experience that older adults are as different as snowflakes; no two are exactly alike.

It is common knowledge that America's older adult population, defined as people ages 65 and older, is growing at record rates. What was referred to years ago as the *age wave* has recently been coined the *Silver Tsunami*. Numbering 37.9 million in 2007, the older adult population is projected to reach 71 million in 2030, an increase of more than 85%.[43] And, to many people's surprise, the fastest growing segment of our population is people age 85 years and older, also known as the *"oldest old."* [44]

According to the National Center for Health Statistics, the average life expectancy is on the rise. In 1900, 1950 and 2000, the average life expectancies were 47.3 years, 68.2 years, and 77.0 years respectively. Just recently, the CDC reported in a press release *"U.S. life expectancy reached nearly 78 year (77.9) ...".*[45] The figures for 2007 indicate life expectancy to be as follows:

Race & Gender	Avg. Life Expectancy
White males	75.8 years
Black males	70.2 years
White female	80.7 years
Black females	77.0 years

While there seems to be awareness of the *statistics* about older adults, there continues to be confusion about the *implications* of the aging process on older adults, families, communities, government and more. As people live longer, the participation of older adults in community services and government programs is expected to increase dramatically and there comes a need to care for those who cannot manage alone. From the various reports I have read over the years, I do believe that activity-level, attitude, connectedness and meaning all play a significant role in both longevity and quality of live.

- Activity-Level – *"It's never too late to exercise."* [46] A Wall Street Journal article entitled *Yes, You Can Turn Back the Clock* referred to a 30-year study which indicated moderate and consistent exercise program, even one started later in life, can have a tremendous effect on aerobic capacity and health. Keep in mind that *activity* does not always equate to *exercise.* In fact, everyday activities that involve getting up and walking or moving around can be quite beneficial. Therefore, engaging in more physical activity today than yesterday can do a body good.

- Attitude – As the saying goes, "*Attitude is everything,*" and it may be more important than many of us realize. "*A 23-year study found that those who had positive perceptions of aging lived an average 7.5 years longer than those with cloudier outlooks.*" [47] According to actor Kirk Douglas, age 91, "*Old age, if you're lucky enough to reach it, is a unique experience in life."* [48] He indicated that humor and the ability to laugh at yourself is an important aspect of life.

- Connectedness – Whether spending time with friends or enjoying the company of a pet, there are emotional and physical health benefits related to the act of bonding. Companionship can help people remain active, have a sense of responsibility, and lessen the feelings of loneliness and isolation that many older adults often experience.

- Meaning – The ability to blend one's sense of past, present and future becomes increasingly important in later life. Having a sense of purpose and reason to get out of bed in the morning can be important for many people. When people have something to look forward to or something to share in their day, there is a tendency to view the world as bigger than one's self. Likewise, if we become preoccupied with ourselves, the focus is often on every little ache, pain, challenge and suspicion over our future fate.

The reason I mention these significant aspects of aging is because it is never too late for older adults, baby boomers and people from other generations to make healthy choices and learn helpful coping strategies.

What Is Normal Aging?

One reason I believe there is so much confusion about the aging process is that common influential images of aging tend to be on the ends of the spectrum. Aging is either portrayed as flattering and idealistic, or it reflects a picture of despair and hopelessness. Whether watching television, seeing a movie on the big screen, selecting a greeting card, or glancing at advertising, you know what I mean.

The positive images portray the *Golden Years* as being joyful and carefree, such as those on assisted living community or supplemental Medicare insurance advertisement show beautiful silver-haired couples walking down the beach at sunset embracing one another or older couples in the park enjoying a picnic lunch with a beautiful wicker basket, fresh cut flowers, and sipping champagne out of fine stemware. They paint the picture that after years of hard work and sacrifice; you have earned the reward, and the good life is yours to enjoy. On the other end of the spectrum are the jokes about aging and unfavorable images on greeting cards showing dentures, walkers and grumpy old folks, suggesting people are *"over the hill"* at age 40, 50, etc.

In addition to images of aging, there is also a collection of one-liners that tends to get a laugh or pack a punch. For example, *"65 is the new 50"* or the joke *"Have you heard the one about the three ages of a man or woman? Youth, middle age and 'you haven't changed a bit'."* Then there is the senility prayer: *"Grant me the senility to forget the people I never liked anyway, the good fortune to run into the ones I do, and the eyesight to tell the difference."*

While images and jokes certainly do paint one picture of aging, the most powerful influence on what we consider to be *Normal Aging* tends to be our personal experiences with older adults, often grandparents, aunts/uncles and neighbors. Even though the concept of aging tends to be misunderstood, aging is a fact of life that often creeps up on us. Whether facing the reality of turning 50, stepping into retirement at age 65, or becoming a Centenarian, people of all ages have something in common: We all face the uncertainty of tomorrow and the mystery of what a new day will bring our way.

While chronological age (the length of time that has passed since one's birth) is a valid marker for qualifying to join the AARP (age 50) or participate in Medicare (age 65), aging has more to do with how a person lives and functions, as opposed to a person's age in years. I believe that instead of asking, *"How* old?" a much better and more relevant measure of age may be *"How functional?"* In other words, are you able to live each day and socialize to the extent you desire? Also, older adults typically perceive themselves as being and looking younger than their actual age.[49]

So what is considered to be normal aging? Experts in the profession of geriatric medicine suggest that there are four primary predictors of successful aging. They are:

1. Regular physical activity
2. Social engagement
3. Freedom from chronic illness
4. Feeling of self-worth.[50]

While three of the predictors of *success* seem straight forward, there tends to be confusion about what is meant by freedom from chronic illness. To start, I need to clarify that the word chronic means that a health condition can be treated; however, there is no cure. Knowing that most older adults have at least one chronic condition, the words *freedom from* refer to the ability to manage an illness and modify one's lifestyle in order to stay active and engaged.

Other attributes of successful aging that differ between researchers include: Life satisfaction, freedom from disability, high/independent functioning, active engagement with life and positive adaptation.

While researchers offer an important point of view, I believe the best people to ask about aging are the older adults themselves. After all, they are the true experts. Based on a study published in 2004, people aged 65 and older identified what they believed were characteristics of normal or successful aging:

Being able to...

- Take care of themselves until close to their time of death
- Make choices about things that affect how they aged, including diet, exercise and smoking
- Cope with the challenges of their later years
- Act according to their inner standards and values
- Meet all of their needs and some of their wants
- Successfully manage chronic disease(s)
- Have friends and family who are there for them
- Feel good about themselves
- Feel satisfied with their lives the majority of the time
- Stay involved with the world and people around them
- Adjust to changes that are related to aging
- Not feel lonely or isolated.[51]

Knowing that aging is a unique experience shaped by many influences in a person's lifetime, what might be considered success is really in the eye of the beholder. For example, based on a scale of 1 to 10, with 10 being the highest, how would you rate your overall wellness and quality of life? If you're like most people I speak with, and assuming you have no disabling health problems, you would probably answer with an eight or nine.

If I were then to ask how your rating would change if you had a life-changing illness, you would probably drop to a four, five or six.

What I find fascinating is that older adults who have a chronic or life-changing medical condition seem to adjust the scale rather than lower their rating. When older adults were recently surveyed about their medical and psychological health, they rated themselves as 8.4 on a scale of 1 to 10 as successful agers, despite illness and disability! What is amazing is that many participants had illnesses often associated with *sick* old people, such as cancer, heart disease and diabetes. In addition, 25% had mental health problems. The authors concluded that optimism and effective coping styles are perhaps more important than other measures, such as health and wellness. Moreover, the best indicator of aging successfully was not physical health, but attitude.[52]

In terms of the supposed Anti-Aging Industry and the many *Miracle Treatments*, save your money. According to scientist S. Jay Olshansky of the University of Illinois at Chicago, *"Anyone claiming that their product will slow, stop or reverse aging is lying."* [53]

Although many aspects of our health are beyond our control, we can reduce our risk of many problems by eating right, exercising regularly, maintaining a healthy weight, managing stress and having regular check-ups and health screenings. Also, beyond one's physical health, experts encourage people to regularly challenge their brains by reading, doing crossword puzzles or engaging in other mentally and intellectually stimulating exercises.

Natural Age-Related Changes

As many of us baby boomers know all too well, we reach our physical peak in our 20s and early 30s. These are the years that our bodies are the strongest, our senses are the keenest, and our minds are the sharpest. While the sequence of changes is similar, the rate at which we experience physical changes tends to be quite individual, often based on one's lifestyle choices, genetics and environmental factors.

The following excerpt from an e-mail I received a few years ago sums up aging and puts many aspects of day-to-day life into perspective:

Have you ever noticed that when you are of a certain age, everything seems uphill from where you are? Stairs are steeper. Groceries are heavier. And, everything is farther away. Why is it, music is turned up louder and people are speaking more softly? ... Is it just me, or do people seem much younger than I was at the same age? And why is it that the people my own age appear so much older than I am?

With advancing age, older adults can expect to experience a variety of natural physical and cognitive changes. A 2004 Business Week article entitled *Aging Is Becoming So Yesterday* elaborated on how our bodies respond to the aging process and what we can expect. One caption from the story stated, *"The organs of the body suffer myriad indignities as we age, deteriorating in response to genetic signals and the wear and tear of daily life."* [54]

While external and internal changes occur as people age, the external changes are most visible. External changes are the physical changes that affect such things as the hair and skin. For example, as early as age 30 or 40, many of us noticed changes to our hair line, hair color and the thickness of our hair. Our skin began to change, and wrinkles began to appear. Other noticeable changes deal with eyesight, hearing, physical strength, balance and coordination.

Internal changes are also happening. Our bodies become weaker. Our sense of smell diminishes. Our sensitivity to touch and hot/cold temperatures changes, and our ability to taste salty and sour foods fades. If that is not enough, our minds may not be as sharp. We may struggle with people's names or have trouble finding the words to express our thoughts. We process and do things slower, and we are more susceptible to illness.

If you would like to read more about specific age-related changes, refer to our web site (www.Caregiving.CC) – click on

Articles and you will find a link to a series I wrote on the aging process. The series goes into more detail about physical, sensory and cognitive changes. The aging series is also available in podcast format and can be downloaded to and iPod or other MP3 player.

As people age, I believe it is important to recognize potential concerns about ability, mobility, safety and vanity.

- Ability – Whether due to natural aging, illness or disease, it is important to recognize if loved one's abilities are limiting their functional independence and mobility. Often, many older adults' struggles with daily living activities are the result of a medical condition. According to the Centers for Disease Control and Prevention, over 40% of non-institutionalized older adults reported difficulties with independent living activities, such as driving or managing public transportation, grocery shopping, preparing meals, housekeeping, managing finances and more.[55] In addition to transportation, another aspect of mobility is being able to move about the home, manage steps, stand up and sit down. Many different medical conditions can affect mobility, such as diabetes (which can result in less feeling in the feet and toes and diminished vision), Parkinson's (with tremors that can lead to instability), and stroke (causing changes in gait, balance, and functional ability).

- Safety – Many aspects of aging can pose safety concerns. For example, the inability to hear an emergency vehicle or car horn while driving, smell smoke or spoiled food and see things clearly and in less than optimal lighting can put older adults in harms way. Diminished hearing and reduced muscle strength can pose challenges in terms of balance, equilibrium, managing steps, controlling a vehicle and more. In addition, as bones become more brittle, a fall or automobile accident could lead to broken bones, serious injury and even death. Changes in the ability to taste and enjoy food can lead to poor nutrition. Cognitive changes can affect judgment, decision-making, logic and more.

- Vanity – Living in a society where youth is revered and aging is denied, many people place value on their physical appearance. Many noticeable differences such as changes to the hair and skin lead people to pursue hair coloring, hair replacement, a toupee or wig, a face lift, lotions and other treatments. In addition to pursuing products and services for mostly cosmetic purposes, many people may also forego using assistive devices such as hearing aids, bifocals, a cane or a walker because they feel self-conscious and conspicuous. Any concerns or embarrassment that affect a person's outward appearance may cause them to venture out into public less, which often leads to isolation. When older adults become less socially active, there is an increased risk of self-neglect, as well as abuse, exploitation and mistreatment from others.

Medical Diagnosis vs. Prognosis

Knowing that most older adults have at least one chronic condition, I believe care must address the whole person, recognizing body, mind and spirit. An article from The Wall Street Journal entitled *Treating an Illness Is One Thing. What About a Patient With Many?* indicated that 66% of people age 65 and older, and 75% of people age 80 and older have multiple chronic health conditions, yet hospitals, clinics and medical research tend to focus primarily on individual health problems. *"The default position is to treat complicated patients as collections of malfunctioning body parts rather than as whole human beings."* [56]

In order to provide the care and support people need and deserve, it is important to understand and distinguish between a few commonly used terms that are often misunderstood.

- Diagnosis – The diagnosis is the identification of a medical condition by its symptoms and placing a name or label on the person's condition. For example, *"Mrs. Smith is showing early stages of Alzheimer's."* People who concentrate on the diagnosis tend to focus on the illness or disease, treatment options and how to manage the condition rather than how the condition affects the person's daily life.

- Morbidity – The term morbidity refers to the prevalence rate of a disease. Co-morbidity or multimorbidity refers to the presence of one or more diseases in addition to the primary disease. Illnesses that are prevalent among older adults include heart disease, cancer, stroke, lower respiratory disease (e.g., chronic obstructive pulmonary disease or COPD), diabetes, Alzheimer's disease, influenza/pneumonia and injury (e.g., motor vehicle, falls).[57]

- Prognosis – The prognosis refers to the prospect of recovery, the anticipated progression of the diagnosed condition, and how the condition is likely to impact a person's physical and cognitive functionality and lifestyle. What type of assistance will they need? People who concentrate on the prognosis tend to focus more on the person, his or her needs and quality of life.

While it is important to be familiar with a medical diagnosis, whether a single health condition or multimorbidity, I believe the purpose of knowing and understanding a diagnosis is to gain insight about the prognosis and the illness' effect on the person. For example, if someone has arthritis, we may know that it leads to pain, swelling and stiffness in the joints. But do we really know how arthritis affects daily living? Disabling diseases, like arthritis which affects 47% of America's older adults, often result in activity limitations, making it increasingly difficult to remain mobile and socially engaged.[58]

From all the people I have talked to over the years, I doubt that most family members (caregivers) really understand the disease of arthritis. Assuming a loved one's arthritis predominately affects the hands, one of the best ways to gain insight is to simulate hand restrictions. For example, you might tape a popsicle stick to one finger, or put band aids around your knuckles to restrict movement. You might even put a thick rubber band around your fingers and thumb. This will help to increase your awareness of all things that require the dexterity and strength of your hands and fingers. You will quickly discover that everything from personal hygiene, using the bathroom, and getting dressed, to preparing and eating meals, managing the mail and paying bills, can be both challenging and frustrating.

Medication Management

As a result of aging and illness, many older adults are taking multiple prescription drugs, over-the-counter medications, supplemental and herbal remedies. According to the book *The Essential Guide to Chronic Illness*, on average, older adults are taking 4½ pills at a time, with some people taking as many as 10 or 12.[59]

Medications are a blessing and a curse. Although many people are healthier because of the availability of prescription drugs, there is a far greater chance for a person to experience adverse reactions as they take more medications for more conditions. Because of the many specialists who could be prescribing a medication, it is critically important to keep a running list of all the medications (over-the-counter, prescription and supplemental) a person is taking. Also include the frequency, dosage and prescribing doctor, and take the list with you to all medical appointments. If that is not convenient, put medicine containers in a bag and take them with you as the labels provide the needed information.

Ideally you will want to help a loved one avoid taking multiple medicines that address similar conditions, being over- or under-stimulated, and combining drugs that do not work well together. For more information on medication safety visit www.Caregiving.CC – click on *Articles* and then *Medication Safety*.

For my mother, during the last six months of her life, she was on so many medications (at a cost of more than $1,000 per month) that it was like she was eating a three-course meal. Because so many doctors and medications were involved in her care, there came a point when the medications were not producing the desired effect. In collaboration with our mom's doctor, we made the decision to take her off her medications and re-introduce them one at a time to find out which one(s) were causing the problem. When her medications were not right, her discomfort was evident, which was unfortunate.

Be aware that vision can also present challenges in terms of refilling prescriptions, sorting and dispensing medications. Pill containers are usually small and the writing on the bottle can be difficult to read. It is best not to have someone identify medications by color alone. Some people may require assistance preparing medicines so they know what to take and when.

Insight And Information – Disease

According to the CDC, *"Currently, about 80% of older adults have at least one chronic condition, and 50% have at least two. ... Among the most frequently occurring conditions in older persons in 2004-05 were: hypertension (48%), diagnosed arthritis (47%), all types of heart disease (32%), any cancer (20%), diabetes (16%) ..."*[60] Other health concerns that are relatively common among older adults include Alzheimer's, respiratory disease (e.g., COPD), influenza/ pneumonia, and injury (both unintentional and intentional).

When a medical condition is diagnosed and/or the need to provide care becomes apparent, it is often the responsibility of family to step up and provide the appropriate types of support. It is at this time that many caregivers discover that they do not know what to do or how best to help. Keep in mind that many people diagnosed with a chronic illness are able to successfully manage their condition and lead an active and productive life.

In your effort to learn about a medical condition, I suggest consulting with a physician or other health care professionals and asking for specific advice and direction. While your parent's physician should be able and willing to point you in the right direction, do not count on him or her to share all that you will need to know and understand due to time constraints. On average, older adults may only spend a total of one hour a year with their primary care physician. According to the Administration on Aging, older adults ages 65 to 74 averaged 6.5 office visits in 2005 compared to 7.7 office visits for those ages 75 and older.[61] Knowing that the time with the doctor averages 7 to 10 minutes per visit, it is not reasonable to expect that detailed information will be shared.

Also, based on research on adult learning, we know that adults retain and are able to recall only about 10-15% of what they hear.[62] Therefore, if a loved one has a serious health condition it becomes essential to go with him or her to medical appointments. A second set of ears can be helpful and may hear and understand things that our elders might not actually hear or want to hear.

Even in the hospital and as part of the discharge process, do not expect to be told all you need or want to know. After all, the average length of stay in acute care hospital is 5.5 days and many people are so distraught or unprepared that they are not ready to hear about restrictions or future care needs, as they are focused on the *"here and now."* [63]

Even after a heart attack, it is quite common that patients leave the hospital with only a couple of prescriptions and a few aspirin. The following excerpt from a Los Angeles Times article entitled *Getting On With Life After A Heart Attack* sums up the reality for many people following discharge. *"They [patients being dischared] receive very little training and education in how to eat, exercise, manage stress and otherwise pick up their lives and care for their damaged tickers."* [64]

In addition to talking with your doctor, it may be helpful to talk to someone who has experienced what you are going through. In addition, I recommend contacting the appropriate national organization for information and learning about resources and support services available in your area. I have listed, in alphabetical order, medical conditions commonly associated with older adults and contact information for the respective national organization(s):

- Alzheimer's (*also see Dementia*) – Refers to a brain disorder that leads to memory gaps and deficits in cognitive function and more. Alzheimer's disease (AD) is the most common form of dementia among older people.

- Arthritis – Refers to a medical condition that causes inflammation, stiffness and pain in the joints. The two most common types of arthritis are osteoarthritis and rheumatoid arthritis.
  - Arthritis Foundation, www.arthritis.org, 800-283-7800

- Cancer – Refers to a group of many related diseases all of which involve out-of-control growth and spread of abnormal cells in any of the body's tissues.
  - American Cancer Society, www.cancer.org, 800-227-2345

- o Leukemia & Lymphoma Society, www.leukemia.org, 800-955-4572

- Cardiovascular Disease – These are diseases that affect the flow of blood throughout the body, including conditions such as an aneurysm, stroke and congestive heart failure.
  - o American Heart Association, www.americanheart.org, 800-242-8721
  - o American Stroke Association, www.americanstroke.com, 800-242-8721
  - o National Stroke Association, www.stroke.org, 800-787-6537

- Dementia – Refers to various disorders that affect the functioning of one's brain, and is characterized by mental decline and impairment. The three chronic health conditions associated with dementia are Alzheimer's (cognitive decline), Parkinson's – (neurologic disorder that affects the central nervous system), and Multi-Infarct Dementia (vascular disease).
  - o Alzheimer's Association, www.alz.org, 800-272-3900 (24-hour helpline)
  - o National Mental Health Association, www.nmha.org, 800-969-6642

- Diabetes – Refers to when the body does not process sugar in the blood stream and often affects circulation and sensitivity in the feet and toes, and also vision.
  - o American Diabetes Association, www.diabetes.org, 800-342-2383

- Huntington's Disease – Refers to a degenerative brain disorder often characterized by uncontrolled movements or tremors, and slowly reduces an individual's ability to walk, think, talk and reason.

- o Huntington's Disease Society of America, www.hdsa.org, 800-345-4372

- Multiple Sclerosis – Refers to a disease that attacks the central nervous system and affects communication between the brain and spinal cord.
  - o National Multiple Sclerosis Society, www.naitonalmssociety.org, 800-344-4867

- Osteoporosis – Refers to a disease that leads to reduced bone density and causes people, especially older women, to be more prone to bone fractures.
  - o National Osteoporosis Foundation, www.nof.org, 202-223-2226

- Parkinson's – Refers to a degenerative neurologic disorder of the central nervous system that impairs motor skills, speech and other functions.
  - o Parkinson's Disease Foundation, www.pdf.org, 800-457-6676

The saying, *"Walk a mile in my shoes,"* suggests that unless you have experienced what someone else is going through, you do not understand and cannot appreciate what the other person is experiencing and feeling. To better understand a loved one's medical condition and provide the appropriate type of support, it can be extremely helpful for caregivers to ponder the following question: How might aging, a fall, a life-changing illness, or the hospitalization or death of a spouse affect the things you do on a day-to-day basis?

Perspective is vital. If we really think about it, chances are we might be able to gain a glimpse of what life is like for our loved ones. Whenever possible, I suggest trying to simulate what it is like for the other person. For example, if a loved one is hard of hearing, put cotton in your ears for an hour to glimpse what it must be like. If someone has deteriorating vision or a disease of the eye, put Vaseline on your glasses or a dot in the middle of each lens. To simulate stroke, assume that one side of your body is lame or not fully functional. Now try going through the day using only your left arm, hand and leg. Dragging your right leg can give you a better idea of what it's like.

If you understand how a medical condition is likely to impact a person's life, it becomes easier to recognize the activities of daily living which your loved one may find challenging. Realizing the limitations a person is likely to face is essential to providing the appropriate care and support. For example, you might want to consider how a medical condition is likely to affect the following:

1. Anxiety and activity levels
2. Hearing and vision
3. Logic, judgment and reasoning
4. Decision-making capability
5. Mental capacity and memory
6. Mobility and reflexes
7. Physical strength and coordination

The point is that a person with a mind-altering condition like dementia is likely to struggle with different issues than a person with cancer who may be experiencing extreme fatigue.

Whether challenges are primarily physical or psychological, many older adults will need assistance with their day-to-day affairs. The alternative is that people do not get the assistance they need and struggle unnecessarily. So, it is only reasonable that as loved ones age or become ill, family members should consider competency issues such as the ability to:

- Care for self
- Focus on a particular activity
- Handle personal affairs and finances

- Live independently
- Manage transportation
- (Re)Fill, sort and take medications as directed
- Demonstrate sound judgment
- Identify potentially dangerous situations

Lifestyle Choices vs. Genetics

There has been a long-standing debate about which has the most impact on the way people age – Nature or Nurture. The Nature theory suggests that certain age-related changes are inevitable and based on genetics – there is little we can do to alter the course. The Nurture theory suggests that lifestyle choices and our environment play the bigger part on our life's course.

According to the CDC, *"Successful aging is largely determined by individual lifestyle choices and not by genetic inheritance."* [65] It estimates 70% of functional limitations or disabilities attributed to the aging process are the result of our own unhealthy decisions and behaviors, including smoking, poor nutrition and a sedentary lifestyle. As the saying goes, *"An ounce of prevention is worth a pound of cure."* In a recent study of well elderly or *"Wellderly,"* researchers found that *"people who exercise regularly, do not smoke, limit their alcohol intake and eat five servings of fruits and vegetables a day live, on average, 14 years longer than people who do not."* [66]

In 2009, the Robert Wood Johnson Foundation reported that, *"Americans overall are not nearly as healthy as they should be, regardless of where they live, their income, education, or racial or ethnic group."* [67]

The key to wellness and living a longer life is prevention by helping people make healthy decisions. *"For too long, we have focused on medical care as the solution to our health problems, when the evidence tells us the opposite," said RWJF president and CEO Risa Lavizzo-Mourey."* [68] In fact, medical care accounted for between 10-15% of preventable early deaths. Lifestyle choices and environmental factors were found to be primary factors indicating how well Americans live.

In addition to the health benefits of avoiding or reducing the affects of illness, there are significant financial benefits. For example, did you know that older adults have more chronic conditions, hospital admissions, doctor and ER visits, and expenditures for prescription drugs than younger age groups.[69] In fact, in 2000, people age 65 and older comprised about 12% of the U.S. population, yet they accounted for about 35% of all hospital stays.[70]

I have no doubt that in an ideal world, prevention through the promotion of wellness and healthy living would be the focus. The problem is that we do not live in an ideal world. Instead, we live in the real world, and if eating better and sticking to an exercise routine were easy, everyone would be doing it.

Therefore, we need to be realistic and optimistic. Also, we know that medical students do not go to medical school to study healthy people. Instead, they focus on disease, diagnosis and treatment. For America's older population, it may be a good thing that medicine is the focus, as opposed to wellness. While we cannot change the past, we can learn from our lifestyle choices and do our best to make our loved ones comfortable as they age.

Health And Wellness

Due to advances in medical technology, people are living longer than ever before. According to the CDC, *"In 2006, persons reaching age 65 had an average life expectancy of an additional 19.0 years (20.3 years for females and 17.4 years for males)."* [71]

While longevity continues to increase, it cannot be the sole focus. As John F. Kennedy once said, *"It is not enough for a great nation merely to have added new years to life. Our objective must also be to add life to those years."*

While it is important for all adults to be aware of their family's health history, there are often choices and changes that can help people avoid health problems or at least delay the onset.

To get an idea of what you might expect in terms of life span, I suggest you consider how other members of your family have aged. Is there a pattern of your parent's genealogy and health history that might suggest a certain medical condition or life expectancy?

For example, Bob Hope's father lived to be 99, suggesting that Hope was likely to live a long life. He died at the age of 100. In the case of David Letterman, it was probably no surprise when he underwent emergency quintuple heart bypass surgery in January of 2000 at the age of 52. Why? Because, his family had a history of heart disease, and his father died of a heart attack in his 50s.

For that reason, life insurance agencies ask applicants about their parents' health history because it is one of the best predictors of the health and wellbeing of the children. If your parents immediate family members have aged similarly, your parent is likely to age in the same way.

For example, on my mother's side of the family, cancer was a concern and neither grandparent lived past their early 70s. This held true for their children – my mom and her siblings. On my father's side, his relatives tended to live into their late 70s and early 80s. The same held true for my father.

There are two fundamental aspects of health. Medicine focuses on cure and treatment, whereas wellness focuses on prevention. When people think of wellness, many think of diet, exercise and other lifestyle choices that may lead to better health. It is estimated that more than 75% of wellness activities focus on physical aspects; however, there are multiple dimensions of wellness, all of which merit attention.

Regardless of one's age, the best medicine may be recognizing and addressing the various dimensions of wellness made popular by Dr. Bill Hettler. The way Dr. Hettler came to establish the *Six Dimensions of Wellness* is a fascinating human interest story. He was first introduced to the topic of wellness and health promotion in May of 1969 during the commencement exercise at his graduation from the University of Cincinnati College of Medicine.

The person offering the commencement address was a professor of Preventive Medicine, someone that most of the students had not seen before as his specialty had very little presence in the medical school curriculum. The speaker began by saying, "*You will save more lives and alleviate more suffering if you never enter the practice of medicine.*" He went on to say that if they "*spent their time helping people learn how to live instead of practicing traditional medicine, they would indeed save more lives and alleviate more suffering.*" [72]

Over the years of practicing medicine, Dr. Hettler realized that peoples' lifestyle choices have a much greater impact on their chances of survival than anything physicians are likely to accomplish. For additional information on Dr. Hettler, visit his website at www.Hettler.com/sixdimen.htm. According to Dr. Hettler, the six dimensions are as follows:

1. Emotional Wellness – refers to one's awareness and acceptance of his/her feelings. An emotionally well person tends to be positive, able to express him/herself appropriately and constructively, enjoy satisfying relationships with others, and cope effectively with stress.

2. Intellectual Wellness – encourages creativity and stimulating one's mind or mental capacity to maintain and expand one's knowledge and skills.

3. Occupational Wellness – involves achieving personal satisfaction and enrichment from one's hobbies and vocation (whether paid or volunteer), and using skills and talents in ways that are meaningful and rewarding.

4. Physical Wellness – encourages activities that develop and maintain one's physical health with regular medical check-ups, self-care, physical exercise, proper nutrition, and the avoidance of tobacco, drugs and excessive alcohol.

5. Social (Interpersonal) Wellness – fosters a positive self-image and encourages positive and frequent interactions in family and community that enable a person to express him or herself, be blessed by others and be a blessing to others.

6. Spiritual Wellness – involves seeking and recognizing meaning in one's life and a spiritually centered belief system that leads to peace, harmony and purpose.

While Dr. Hettler focuses on six dimensions of wellness, others believe that there are other important dimensions such as environmental wellness and financial wellness.

- Environmental Wellness – refers to a lifestyle that is respectful of nature and leads people to conserve energy and to be environmentally conscious and considerate.

- Financial Wellness – refers to having an understanding of one's financial situation and sufficient resources to meet needs and some wants.

Graphical depictions of the Wellness model often show each factor as a piece of a pie. I personally view the wellness model as a teeter-totter because it reflects balance and change. If one aspect of wellness is reduced, the other dimensions often become more important to maintain balance and achieve a desired quality of life.

A Closing Thought

Aging is a unique experience, and it is incorrect and potentially harmful to stereotype older adults as being all the same. It is equally inaccurate and inappropriate to accept the predominate declinist assumption that aging is all about loss. Many people fear aging like they fear wrinkles and other physical indicators often associated with aging.

One of my favorite advertisements is for SunRise Assisted Living communities from 2002. The ad features a photo of an elderly lady's wrinkly face with the headline *"Every line tells a story,"* referring to the lines on her face. The wording went on to say *"Every hard-earned line is a legacy and a lesson to us all."* What a great perspective and outlook on life.

George Valliant, author of the book *Aging Well*, indicates successful aging means *"giving to others joyously whenever one is able, and receiving from others gratefully whenever one needs it."* [73] I believe the idea of *normal, successful* or *graceful* aging is the ability to do all you want without being limited by disease, lack of energy, or lack of financial resources.

My question to you is this: What do *you* consider to be normal or successful aging? I encourage you to take time and reflect on the aspects of aging that are most important to you and your family members. Doing so can help you:

1. Understand a loved one's values, personal beliefs and ideals related to the aging process.

2. Determine your health goals and priorities for the later years of life.

3. Communicate your personal preferences should you find yourself in need of care or assistance.

It is much easier for family, friends and health care professionals to carry out someone's wishes when they know what they are. Therefore, we encourage people to write down and share their wishes with those who may be called upon to provide care or make decisions on their behalf.

If you have concerns about yourself or a loved one's health, wellbeing or quality of life, speak with a physician or other health care professionals to determine what type of treatment, care and support may be appropriate.

The more frequently you see your loved ones, the more difficult it tends to be to recognize or come to grips with the changes commonly associated with aging. Think about it. Changes are more obvious if you have not seen someone in a long time.

Regardless of how often you see someone, most people are unable to distinguish between normal aging and conditions that may be a cause for concern. I hope the information shared in this chapter gives you an idea of what to expect, and helps you know what type of support is most appropriate and how to provide it. Also, I hope it encourages you to cherish relationships.

KEY LEARNINGS – *Top three findings from this chapter:*
1.
2.
3.

ACTION ITEMS - *Things you want to do or do differently:*		
Check when Completed	*Action Item*	*Target Completion Date*

"People do not care how much you know,
until they know how much you care."
– Unknown

4.

The Care Receiver Perspective

Often we do not understand life from another person's perspective because we lack experience. To help clarify this concept, imagine what it would be like if you were to lose the ability or privilege to drive or get around town. When I am left without a car after I have taken it in to be serviced, the thought of not having the freedom or ability to drive creates anxiety, even if I have no need go out or plans to be somewhere. What would it be like for you if you had to rely on others for transportation to go shopping, visit family or friends, attend religious services, go out for dinner or see a movie?

Frankly, I question if we can really understand life from the perspective of an older adult or a person with a chronic or life-threatening illness without confronting a similar situation. What do you think? Can you imagine and understand what it must be like to go through life with diminished vision, poor hearing, a lack of energy, etc.? In addition to facing what might be considered normal age-related changes, imagine what it would be like to be diagnosed and living with one or more chronic medical condition. We will explore these issues and more in this chapter.

The USA Today newspaper often runs Snapshots® that catch my eye. Two in particular that were insightful are:

- *What is your greatest fear about retirement?* The top three responses were: High health care costs (28%), Running out of money (24%), and Inability to maintain standard of living (18%) [74]

- *Our greatest fears about getting old.* The top three responses were: "Health problems" (32%), "Income problems" (19%) and "Being dependent" (8%).

Also insightful is a poem entitled *Look Closer, See Me*. Years ago, when an old woman died in the geriatric ward of a small hospital in Scotland, it was believed she had nothing left of any value. Later, when the nurses were going through her belongings, they found the following poem which shares the importance of seeing a person for who he or she is, not simply how one appears. The woman is now known as Anonymous.

Look Closer, *See Me*

What do you see, people, what do you see?
What are you thinking, when you look at me?
A crabby old woman, not very wise.
Uncertain of habit, with far-away eyes,
Who dribbles her food and makes no reply.
When you say in a loud voice "I do wish you'd try!"

Who seems not to notice the things that you do.
And forever is losing a stocking or shoe.
Who, unresisting or not; lets you do as you will.
With bathing and feeding, the long day to fill.
Is that what you're thinking, is that what you see?
Then open your eyes, you're not looking at me.

I'll tell you who I am as I sit here so still!
As I rise at your bidding, as I eat at your will.
I'm a small child of 10 with a father and mother,
brothers and sisters, who loved one another.
A young girl of 16 with wings on her feet,
dreaming that soon now a lover she'll meet.

A bride soon at 20 — my heart gives a leap,
Remembering the vows that I promised to keep.
At 25 now I have young of my own
Who need me to build a secure happy home.
A woman of 30, my young now grow fast,
Bound to each other with ties that should last.

At 40, my young sons have grown and are gone,
But my man's beside me to see I do not mourn.
At 50 once more babies play around my knee,
Again we know children, my loved one and me.
Dark days are upon me, my husband is dead,
I look at the future, I shudder with dread.

For my young are all rearing young of their own.
And I think of the years and the love that I've known.
I'm an old woman now and nature is cruel,
'Tis her jest to make old age look like a fool.
The body is crumbled, grace and vigor depart.
There is now a stone where I once had a heart.
But inside this old carcass, a young girl still dwells,
And now and again my battered heart swells.
I remember the joy, I remember the pain,
And I'm loving and living life over again.
I think of the years all too few — gone too fast,
And accept the stark fact that nothing can last.
So open your eyes, people, open and see.
Not a crabby old woman, LOOK CLOSER, SEE ME.

Ask The Experts

One of the best ways to gain insight on aging is to ask the experts. After all, who knows the topic better than people who are older than 65? Since January 2007, I have had the privilege to teach a graduate level course on aging and adult development at the University of Cincinnati. Most of my students are majoring in health education and have very little experience interacting or working with older adults. Knowing the power of perspective, the first project I assign requires them to interview an older adult and write about their discoveries and observations. A few of the questions they are instructed to ask and some of what I believe are revealing answers follow.

With the permission of my students from whose papers I have extracted snippets, I share a few of the responses for the benefit of understanding perspectives that are often overlooked or misunderstood.

Perspective vs. Reality of Aging – How is aging consistent with, or different from, what the person expected?

- "Anyone who said old age is your golden years is a damn fool. This whole notion of walking along the beach and playing with grandkids is perception, but not reality. You lose family. You lose friends who have become family. Frankly, that has been devastating because they know, appreciate and understand you — one thing I've found that my children do not."

- "It seems like one day I woke up and everything was harder; you cannot dress yourself, put on shoes and socks, it takes longer to shower, cook, eat, clean and walk places."

- "When you get older you have to develop patience because everything takes longer. I never expected it would take so much longer to do simple things I've done all my life."

- "Time goes by so quickly. All of a sudden I'm elderly. I do not feel elderly, however, I am and it is what it is."

- "I never imagined getting old alone. I wish I would have taken the time to maintain friendships, get involved in activities and meet new people. It's been so long since I had a social circle, and frankly, I'm lonely."

- "I never knew that having major illness will be so financially draining. Because of my illness and the apparent burden I am to my wife and kids, I feel as though resentment is a big part of my frustration. I feel certain that they blame me and believe that my current situation is due to poor or unhealthy choices I've made in my life. "

- "I thought I would be in better health, and frankly, I am dismayed that I have so many things going wrong. I was always a capable and self-sufficient person, but now that my vision is almost gone and I am practically disabled, I am totally dependent on others, which is hard."

Challenges and Frustrations – What are the person's top three or four health concerns?

- "I've been doing things my own way for so long that my family sees me as being bossy or crabby when I want things done a certain way. I am resistant to change, but I'm not this mean person that my kids make me out to be."

- "My biggest complaint about aging is my lack of energy. I get tired so quickly, and I just cannot go at the pace younger people move at."

- "The inability to drive was one of the hardest obstacles I've ever faced."

- "Giving up my weekly golf (due to vision limitations) was frustrating as it also meant giving up the one social activity I most looked forward to."

- "Worst of all, when you are aging, you have to depend on other people for everything, even with simple things like putting on your socks."

- "I have always kept my house orderly, but now it seems like there are stacks everywhere and I just cannot cope."

- "My biggest frustration is people minimize me because I am older. It seems that everyone from retail clerks to people I see regularly do not take me and the things I say seriously. I just want to be treated like a normal person who is entitled to her opinion and a little bit of dignity and respect."

- "I am very conscious of the lack of respect on the part of the general public, and the general public seems to believe that I need to be talked down to. It's often my experience that those who do not know me assume that I am demented and treat me as though I do not get it."

- "There is a general attitude about older adults; people should not make assumptions about us just because we are gray. I admit that I am old, and I do not see anything wrong with it. It's a fact of life."

- "My biggest concern is my ability to remain independent. I do not want to be a burden to my child."

- "Arthritis is just an annoying pain that you have to deal with."

- "I try to share things now, but it does not seem like my family wants to listen."

- "One of my biggest challenges has been losing my friends as I age. Friends cannot be replaced, so I feel the loss in major ways — ways that younger generations probably cannot understand."

- "Fear of the unknown is a big challenge for me. I would like to know how I will go out, what the light at the end of the tunnel will look like; there are lots of mysteries around the death experience. But, when I die, my aggravations will be over and that provides a lot of comfort to me."

- "My biggest frustration is not being as sharp as I used to be. I hope it is just occasional forgetfulness. I see people I have known for years, and I cannot remember their names. I walk to a room in my house and forget what I was going to get. Privately, it is frustrating beyond belief. Publically, it is downright embarrassing."

Advice and Recommendations – What is the best part about being older, and if the person could share one piece of advice, what would it be?

- "My advice is that you never know what's in store for you so you had better be prepared for anything."

- "You do not have to have such a great memory if you always tell the truth."

- "My advice is to always honor your mother and father, regardless of their age, and remember they are people and they matter. My children tried to get me to move into a retirement home not long after my wife died because they felt I could not care for myself. I was shocked and disappointed that they never asked for my opinion or cared to hear what I thought about the whole situation."

- "We want to make informed decisions, so help us by sharing information and being open to our questions. If you want to influence me, give me the reasons; do not just tell me what I have to do."

- "My advice to younger people is live your life as though each day may be your last and never take anything for granted. And, of course, respect your elders."

- "As we get older, we tend to see how fragile life really is, and we come to realize that we are mortal. Do not let life pass you by. Take time to stop and smell the roses, see the beauty of the things around you, and look for the good in everyone."

In addition to what I consider to be invaluable wisdom and important sound bites to hear and understand, the perspectives of my students are equally fascinating. The following are a few of their comments. My guess is that they will be able to relate to a few of their pearls of wisdom.

Most Significant Insight (of students) – What is the most significant insight or new perspective you gained from speaking with an older person?

- "As I reflected on this project, I came to realize that prior to this conversation I was always the one answering the questions posed by my granddad. Never before could I remember a time when I asked him about what was going on in his life or how he felt about something other than the obligatory, "Is there anything I can do to be helpful?"

- "Grandma has always been the person that people rely on; not the one that has to rely on others. I think that is part of the reason why she finds it so difficult, even demoralizing, to accept support from others. I believe that some of the reasons why she is still alive and kicking are her wit, her stubbornness, her ability to always see the good in other people and her sense of feeling needed."

- "People have always told me that my grandmother was awesome. Until I sat down and actually spoke to her with the purpose of getting to know who she is as a person and learning about her life, I was oblivious to how special and sweet she really is. There were also so many things I really never understood, like how hard it was for her to stop driving, continuing on with life after my grandpa died, etc."

- "I wish my children would have more patience with me. Believe me, if I could do things faster, trust me I would."

- "Frankly I was scared to ask her the questions because I thought they might make her upset. Also, I didn't want to ask her anything that might make her sad or make her feel bad. This was an eye-opening experience for both of us."

- "When I asked her about her challenges and frustrations, I found it interesting that she didn't answer the question as pertaining to herself, but as being an elderly person."

- "I was so surprised; she thinks of herself as a healthy person, yet she has numerous health problems."

- "I realize my grandmother won't be here forever and I really do want to treasure and appreciate the time I do have with her."

- "After concluding my interview, I not only had more of an insight of my grandmother, but I had more insight to where I get some of my core values, and I was disappointed in myself for not knowing this information before."

- "My grandma refuses to surround herself with other people her age or older. Instead, she likes to be around younger people so she does not feel so old."

- "Because of her defiance and stubborn attitude, I'm concerned that others will not tolerate her should she need care in her home or need to move to a nursing home."

As you reflect on your caregiving situation, are you more focused on the person for whom you are caring, or his/her illness and day-to-day issues? My recommendation is to focus on the person and your relationship.

Reactions To A Diagnosis

In addition to sharing perspectives on aging, I believe it is equally important to gain insight on what it must be like for the person who diagnosed with a life-changing illness. For most people their view of life and the world collapses. *"They wrestle to answer questions, such as, 'Why did this happen?' 'Why me?' and 'Who or what is responsible for this?'"* ... *They may even resign to illness being a part of life and aging."* [76]

The following are comments describing the experience of being diagnosed. Listen carefully to the words people used as they offer a glimpse of what it must be like:

* An article entitled *Dropping the Bomb: The experience of Being Diagnosed with Parkinson's Disease* described it this way: *"...receiving the diagnosis of Parkinson's Disease for many people is a life altering experience, shared by the conflicting sentiments of relief and turmoil — relief related to naming the responsible entity and fear related to an ominous forecast for the future ... the impact of PD on one's life is all encompassing ... complete havoc [is] experienced by the participant upon receiving the diagnosis..."* [77]

* *"My world was rocked and everything changed in a matter of minutes. As a result of my stroke I can no longer work or drive. I can no longer dress myself, mop the floor, or manage aspects of life that yesterday I took for granted. It also took away our dreams for retirement as the idea of traveling and sightseeing is out. I'm now dependent, and she's now my caregiver."* [78]

* *"One minute, I'm cutting the grass, the next minute I'm in the back of an ambulance. I had a heart attack. All of a sudden*

my kids who rarely come home or express any interest in me are all here suffocating me, telling me what to do. Why is everyone overreacting and what the 'heck' gives them the right to tell me what to do? If that's not enough, my doctor is now telling me I should not smoke, I need to eat better, exercise, avoid potentially stressful situations and not overdo it. All I want to do is get out of here. And, I want to know how soon I can have sex with my wife." [79]

- *"The doctor came in with a tear in his eye," she recalled. "'It's bad.' Those were his exact words. 'You have maybe six months.'"* [80]

- *"When I found out I had breast cancer ... I became a comedian. Not the kind anyone paid to see. Just the kind ... offering offbeat opinions, wiseacre remarks, outrageous commentary ... I wanted to be someone, a recognizable personality, a full-blooded, memorable human being, and not just a cancer patient. I had already lost the person I used to be, that healthy, energetic 45-year-old woman. I wasn't capable of losing more ... "I feel as if I want to ask you," I told my oncologist, "how to live." She told me I could live as I had before — working, taking care of kids, exercising, traveling, enjoying life. Anything, really. I could lead a normal life."* [81]

Acknowledging A Medical Condition

While celebrities such as Michael J. Fox and Charlton Heston have come forward to publically acknowledge their conditions, people are generally reluctant to announce any type of personal medical challenge. Many people never go public as they do not want to admit they have a medical condition. Others do not go public because they fear they will be treated differently. When a person has a chronic or life-changing illness, regardless of age, it is important to focus on his/her ability, not the disability. As Miss Wheelchair Ohio said,

"I'm a person first, disabled second. That's how I like people to see me. It's OK if you notice the wheelchair, but do not let it define me as a person." [82] The importance of person first is critical to understand. While the difference may seem insignificant, Miss Wheelchair Ohio is a *"person with a disability"* NOT a *"disabled person."* When disabled comes before person, the focus is on the disability and not the person. People want to be defined by their personhood and personality, not by a diagnosis.

Many people also struggle with deciding when and how to let others know. Every day about 1,000 people are diagnosed with Alzheimer's disease. Individuals and their families often suffer in silence until such time as the signs and symptoms become too apparent for others to ignore. A recent Wall Street Journal article indicated that there are many benefits of acknowledging the disease with others. *"If you're not hiding your illness, you'll feel less stress when you forget someone's name or do something odd. Also, you can seek support, and your loved ones can make better use of community resources. If you do not go public there is often needless isolation out of fear."* [83]

The article also told the story of a lady and her personal experience. *"At first, I didn't want to tell anyone, she says. Only her husband knew ... Four months later, when they dropped the Christmas cards in the mailbox, it was both terrifying and a relief."* In the cards, she wrote: *"I have it, I cannot deny it, and I will die of it eventually, but the more people hear about it, the less scary it gets."* [84]

Regardless of a person's illness, people react differently and do things differently. There is no right or wrong way to respond to a diagnosis. For example, some people respond with *Guarded Anticipation*, others with a need for *Becoming Informed, Dealing with Disease Dynamics* and *Negotiating with Mr. [disease]*. [85] Which best describes how your loved ones are most likely to respond?

- Guarded Anticipation — a careful reluctance to accept the diagnosis and not stir up too much anxiety about the future, as a way to protect one's self and others.

- Becoming Informed — a lack of familiarity or knowledge leads to seeking information and learning about an illness from people living with the condition to get personalized insight and be encouraged from what are referred to as parallel comparisons.

- Disease Dynamics — a way of dealing with struggles and the unique aspects of symptoms, medications, therapies and more, resulting from a particular illness.

- Negotiating with Mr. [Disease] — a way of incorporating the reality of a disease into everyday life and referring to the disease by name.

How Illness And Aging Affect People

Aging and illness are more than a biological experience. *"The patient with the [chronic] illness is profoundly affected in the biological, psychological, and social functioning arenas [domains]."* [86]

Biological Domain
- Functional Status — ability to handle/manage daily living activities, recreation and personal care. [87]
- Physical Symptoms — symptoms and side effects from treatment, continually remind of the illness, the sense of being powerless and helpless. [88, 89]

Psychological Domain
- Grief and Sorrow – ensuing grief, loss of bodily function, the person who once was. [90, 91, 92]

- Fears — constant uncertainty, difficulty understanding, adapting to a new regimen and routine, and coping with fears common to people with a chronic illness. Fears include losses such as control, self-image, independence, as well as stigma, abandonment, expression of anger, isolation and death. Also, fears and anxiety about the future, their children's future, and how relationships are likely to be affected by illness.[93]

Economic Domain

- Debilitating illnesses lead to financial drain from health- and care-related costs, inability to work and earn an income.[94]

Social Domain

- Illness often leads to decreased level of participation in social activities and change in relationships. Also, the individual and his/her family and friends may confront and be uncomfortable coping with mortality which is inevitably linked with chronic illness.[95]

The Wooden Bowl

The affects of aging may be inevitable, but they do not lessen the value of human life. Most of us have been told to respect our elders ever since we were children, but what does that really mean? It may be easier to understand the meaning and application of the word respect by first looking at the word disrespect. Disrespect includes ignoring someone's thoughts or feelings, being condescending, being neglectful, forcing your opinion and being rude or selfish. Now consider the opposites.

There is a strong connection between the words honor, obey and respect. As you provide care for your aging parents remember the Golden Rule. *Do unto others as you would have them do to you.* Isn't that really what it is all about? The Wooden Bowl story clearly makes the point:

A frail old man went to live with his son, daughter-in-law and 4-year-old grandson. The old man's hands trembled, his eyesight blurred, and his step faltered. The family ate together at the table, but the elderly Grandfather's shaky hands and failing sight made eating difficult. Peas rolled off the spoon onto the floor. When he grasped the glass, milk spilled on the tablecloth. The son and daughter-in-law became irritated with the mess. "We must do something with Grandpa," said the son. "I have had enough of spilled milk, noisy eating, and food on the floor." So the husband and the wife set a small table in the corner.

There Grandpa ate alone while the rest of the family enjoyed their dinner. Since Grandpa had broken a dish or two, his food was served in a wooden bowl. When the family glanced in Grandpa's direction, sometimes he had a tear in his eye as he sat alone. Still the only words the couple had for him were sharp admonitions when he dropped his fork or spilled food. The 4-year-old watched it all in silence.

One evening before supper, the father noticed his son playing with wood scraps on the floor. He asked the child sweetly, "What are you making?" Just as sweetly the boy responded, "Oh, I am making a little wooden bowl for you to eat your food when you grow old." The 4-year-old smiled and went on with his work.

The words so struck the parents that they were speechless. Then tears started to stream down their cheeks. Though no words were spoken, both knew what must be done. That evening the husband took the Grandfather's hand and gently led him to the family table.

For the remainder of his days he ate every meal with the family. For some reason, neither the husband nor wife seemed to care any longer when a fork dropped, milk spilled, or the tablecloth soiled. – Anonymous

Other Ways To Gain Insight

While not everyone is willing to open up, share their concerns and talk freely about functional concerns or fears that may be used against them to try and force change, the best way to gain insight is to sit down and talk with one another. I will bet you will find that some people are scared about diminishing mental and physical abilities, concerned about being a burden to family, or are fearful of dying. A person may prefer to ignore the facts, be unwilling to admit they are part of a demographic group (e.g., senior citizens), or may fear losing their independence. Many older adults, especially those who have lived through the Great Depression, may fear spending money or be concerned about depleting their life savings. People may also fear the future or fear loneliness. The list goes on and on. When you try to figure out why a person acts the way they do, think about what might be going through their mind. Talk and ask questions.

Another great way to gain perspective is to watch movies. There are a number of classics and also newer movies that offer a glimpse of reality. A few movies I highly recommend include *On Golden Pond, Driving Miss Daisy, Dad, The Notebook, Cocoon, Marvin's Room, To Dance with the White Dog, The Bucket List* and *The Curious Case of Benjamin Button and UP* (Disney Pixar's 2009 release).

Mirror, Mirror On The Wall

I have vivid memories of touring retirement communities with my parents in the mid-90s. One of the comments I was surprised by was when my dad said *"Look at all these old people."* It came as a surprise because he was probably five to 10 years older that most of the residents. What I did not realize at the time is that it is apparently quite common for older people to feel younger that their numeric age — about 13 years younger, in fact.[96] In addition to perceived age, older adults also indicated they looked considerably younger, about 10 years than their chronological age. Based on this information it is no wonder why many older adults view their situation more favorably than their adult children.

Besides the advertisements and images that make retire-ment look glamorous, elderly people themselves seem to deny aging in many other ways. Our society is so wrapped up in cosmetic surgery miracles, hair alterations and sexual performance enhancers, that much of our culture no longer acknowledges aging, or even understands how to identify the aging process when it is happening right under our noses.

People young and old have a difficult time coping with the reality of aging. A Dear Abby column, entitled *Dad's Alzheimer Diagnosis is Meet by Angry Siblings' Denial* indicates the common struggles and thinking people often face.

> *"For years now, my dad's health has slowly deteriorated. He has good days when he kind of knows what's going on, and bad days when his whole world is off balance. Recently, he suffered some min-strokes, and last September the doctor diagnosed him with Alzheimer's.*
>
> *I was there when Dad was diagnosed. You could see the look of relief on his face to finally have a name for what was going on inside him. He told the doctor, "Well at least now I know I'm not going crazy."*
>
> *The problem is his siblings. They get angry at Mom when she tells the doctor how Dad is at home and accuse her of exaggerating. They get upset with us for not letting Dad*

drive, even though he does not see well and has been known to get lost. They have even gone behind out backs and told Dad he does not have Alzheimer's, which only compounds the problem.

... Poor mom has a hard enough time being a caregiver to a man who does not always recognize us and cannot remember names."

RESPONSE: ...Your father's siblings are in deep denial – which is probably why they cannot bring themselves to admit what is really happening. Their anger at your mother is part of their denial. They would rather believe that she is exaggerating than come to grips with the truth ... " [97]

Do not be surprised if your loved ones, siblings, relatives and/or friends are in denial about what you believe may be quite apparent. Denial is a coping mechanism for many, and people cannot be forced to acknowledge something. They may also confuse Alzheimer's with normal aging.

According to a SNAPSHOT® from USA Today entitled *Alzheimer's often confused with aging*, it is often one year after people experience symptoms until they get medical attention. Caregivers indicated the following reasons for the delay: *fear of diagnosis (9%), denial (31%), confusion with normal signs of aging (57%)."* [98] Although the information is specific to a study on Alzheimer's, I believe the findings are relevant regardless of the disease.

If family or friends are in denial, my recommendation is to share information over time that might help them recognize what may seem obvious to you. Also, be careful not to enable. For example, if a loved one indicates everything is okay, do not come to their rescue so quickly. Assuming that safety is not a concern, it may be good to let them struggle a bit in hopes they might be more willing to acknowledge their limitations and be more accepting of assistance. Reassure them that you are there to help if and when they need it.

Care Sharing

One of the challenges with the terms caregiving and care receiving is that it makes the caring process seem lopsided, as though one person is giving, which implies he or she is not receiving, and visa versa. A common phrase I often hear is that it is easier to give than to receive. In fact, many people who have been self-sufficient their entire life, find it hard to accept the kind gestures of others. So, rather than using the terms giving and receiving, I encourage people to think of it as sharing. I believe the term *care sharing* better represents the care experience than caregiving because it more accurately reflects a mutual benefit. In addition to being stated more positively, it is also more representative of the care process and implies everyone involved in the process has something to gain.

As people face functional challenges due to age-related health problems, a chronic disease or an injury, it is quite common to hear them say they do not want to be a burden to their family. This type of comment is indicative of the perceived imbalance and lack of benefit to the caregivers. The term caregiving often conjures up thoughts of people scurrying around completing a series of tasks. While there are many tactical activities associated with caregiving, such as providing help with daily living activities including meals, medications, chores and errands, one aspect of the care process that many people overlook is relationship or companionship. Also, if you and your family are, for whatever reason, not able to provide the level of care or support a loved one may need, you might share the responsibility with friends or professional caregivers.

It is important to clarify that *getting* or *accepting* help does not mean someone loses their independence or becomes dependent. Instead, assistance can help people maximize their independence and maintain it for a longer period of time. With the advancements in the long-term care industry over the past 10 years, there are many options, programs and innovations that enable people to maintain their independence. Although nursing homes have long been thought of as the ideal living environment for today's seniors, in fact far fewer live in nursing homes than most people expect. According to the AARP, older adults prefer living at home.[99] It is estimated that just over 1% of people age 65–74 live in a nursing home at any given time. For folks age 75-84, the number is just shy of 5%. And, of those people age 85 and older, greater than 80% either live with family or alone.[100]

Mental Health

In addition to physical health, it is also important to recognize possible mental health concerns. While most of us have probably lost our keys or misplaced something that was under our nose the whole time, a frequent question people have is, *"Is there a reason to be concerned, or might it just be a Senior Moment?"* It is typically a person's short-term memory, or ability to recall recent activities or events that is most often affected. The information stored in our long-term memory, tends to cover a longer span of time, be of greater importance and is referred to more often. In many cases, older people simply need more time to process information as it may take them longer to bring their thoughts to mind or to express themselves. The more complex or involved the process of recalling information, the more disadvantaged an older person is.

If loved ones appear to have lost interest in things they once enjoyed, or if they consistently rely on someone else to make decisions, there may be a reason to be concerned. The term cognitive function refers to a person's mental status and has to do with the human brain. The brain is what enables a person to ride a bike, read a book, laugh at a joke, and know when to eat or go to sleep. Cognitive function involves memory performance, a person's intelligence and the ability to pay attention. Many older adults will face minor memory impairments and slower cognitive processing ability as part of the normal aging process. For healthy older adults, the losses tend to be more annoying than compromising of daily functioning.

It is important to recognize and address behavioral changes when a loved one just does not seem right. Seek medical attention and find out what treatments are available. The Alzheimer's Association indicates that *"As many as 10% of all people 65 years of age and older have Alzheimer's. As many as 50% of all people 85 and older have the disease."* [101]

Dementia, depression and delirium are conditions that often go undiagnosed and untreated. The incidence of all three conditions increases as people age. The challenge is to identify abnormal behavior and to decide when to pursue medical attention. Also, do not overlook the possibility of unusual behavior being the result of substance abuse. While there are many similarities between dementia, depression and delirium, it is important to pursue medical attention and be able to report any and all symptoms to help medical professionals determine the cause and make a diagnosis, so a person can receive appropriate treatment.

Dementia is a term that describes disorders that affect the functioning of one's brain, and is characterized by mental decline and impairment. Dementia and Alzheimer's are two different conditions. Alzheimer's, a degenerative disorder of the brain, is reported to be the most common cause of dementia in older adults. People with Alzheimer's have dementia; however people with dementia do not necessarily have Alzheimer's. For example, people with Parkinson's (a neurological disorder) can have dementia. A common form of dementia is a condition referred to as Multi-Infarct, a vascular disease, where blood flow is cut off from a certain part of the brain (mini-stroke) resulting in permanent damage and associated loss of mental capacity. Dementia is generally progressive and interferes with normal daily activity. Over time, people with dementia lose the ability to function independently.

A person with dementia often has trouble with the ability to recall information, solve problems and speak. People also may act strange or seem moody. Another characteristic is an inability to make decisions or respond to questions. As a result, it is common for a person with dementia to say things like *"That's fine with me,"* or *"I'll have what you're having,"* as they may be unable to process things on their own. As conditions worsen, paranoia, delusions and hallucinations may occur. Alzheimer's is known to progress in stages. A resource that may help you better understand the disease is *Stages of Alzheimer's* from the Alzheimer's Association (www.alz.org/ alzheimers_ disease_stages_of_alzheimers.asp). You might also search their website for *Sundowning*, which is restlessness that often occurs at the end of the day, and *Shadowing*, which is when a person follows or mimics the caregiver, or talks, interrupts and asks questions repeatedly.

Depression refers to a mood disorder that can affect both a person's mind and body. Although many people never seek treatment for depression, those that do often experience improvement. While everyone occasionally feels depressed or sad, depression is characterized by intense sadness that lasts for a period of two weeks or longer, and impacts a person's ability to lead a normal life. Depression that goes untreated can lead to medical complications and even suicide.

According to Hanley-Hazelman, a treatment center for chemical dependency in West Palm Beach, Florida, alcohol is a problem for an estimated eight million older Americans. *"People just do not connect sweet little gray-haired grandmothers with alcoholism, according to the center's director of older adult services. Many people use alcohol and/or sedatives to relieve pain, grief or depression. For many who begin to drink later in life, "The biggest problem is that they have lost a sense of purpose. They do not feel needed anymore,"* according to the Center's Director. [102]

Depression can also be the result of a chronic pain. *"Pain should not be an inevitable part of growing old. An estimated 20-40% of Americans age 65 and older suffer from long-term pain, but only a fraction receives treatment."* [103] The article indicated that medical professionals are working to rename pain problems as *persistent pain*, rather than *chronic pain*, as the word chronic conjures up the notion that nothing can be done to relieve the pain. Many pain conditions can be successfully treated, improving one's functioning and decreasing pain. If you think pain may be a concern, visit the American Geriatrics Society Foundation website for additional information: www.HealthInAging.org/public_education/pain.

Delirium is a disorder, not a disease, which appears suddenly, often within hours or days, and may come and go throughout the day. A person who is delirious may appear disoriented, exhibit varying levels of consciousness, have disorganized speech, and an inability to comprehend what is being said. With delirium, there is typically an underlying cause such as infection, dehydration, physical illness, head injury, trauma, substance abuse or a reaction to medications (e.g. prescription, over-the-counter, supplements).

Delirium can be frightening, as a loved one acts unpredictably, is uncooperative and sometimes acts violently. It is not unusual for a delirious person to have mood swings and appear as if he or she is living in his/her own world. Physical restraints may be needed to prevent a delirious person from harming themselves or others.

If you have concern about cognitive function or behavior changes, or anxiety pursue medical attention and ask about treatments that may be available. To help health care professionals identify the cause and determine the necessary treatment, it is important to report any symptoms.

A Closing Thought

As a caregiver, make sure to give consideration to the care recipient's perspective and feelings. Likewise, if you are a care recipient, give consideration to the caregiver's role. Realize that most people try the do their best and that most everyone has good intentions. It is often how those intentions are communicated or demonstrated that can be challenging. Dealing with older parents can be extremely challenging. This challenge is often magnified because family members usually have no idea how parents are going to react to an expressed concern over their wellbeing and attempts to help.

In addition, do not be surprised if loved ones respond in unexpected ways. For example, I was baffled by the way my father was with money. What I did not realize was that he was used to earning an income all his life and then one day he suddenly made the switch from earning and saving to spending. With spending came the fear of depleting his funds and running out of money.

I have seen many people face similar challenges when they retire. Imagine having worked for 40 or more years and then one day transitioning from work life into a life of retirement. Imagine using skills and abilities on a daily basis and then suddenly stopping. Whether a person worked in a factory or was responsible for directing a team of people, everyone likes to feel as though his or her contributions are important and valuable. When people retire and businesses continue to operate without them, they often question their value. The point is that care recipients often internalize challenges that family members never recognize or acknowledge. Remember to always focus on the *person* first.

KEY LEARNINGS – *Top three findings from this chapter:*
1.
2.
3.

ACTION ITEMS - *Things you want to do or do differently:*

Check when Completed	*Action Item*	*Target Completion Date*

EXERCISE: Gather Personal Information

As a caregiver, you will undoubtedly need access to the care recipient's personal information at a moment's notice. I strongly suggest you capture the following information. For your sake, <u>do not</u> skip this exercise and come back to it later. Also, **make sure to protect and keep this information confidential** as it includes a place to list Social Security and Medicare Claim numbers. Therefore, if this information gets into the wrong hands it could be used to steal someone's identity. Only disclose this information to people who have a need to know. NOTE: If you would like to download the exercise, you can do so by visiting our website at www.Caregiving.CC – Click on *Articles* and then *Worksheet — Personal Information*. The worksheet is available in both Microsoft Word and Adobe PDF formats. Keep a hard copy of the worksheet safe and accessible, so you can find it when you need it.

Name (Legal):

Address:

Telephone #'s (home, cell):

Social Security #:

Medicare Claim #:

Place of Employment(*if working*):

Address:

Work Telephone #:

Supervisor's Name:

For each of the following medical professionals, indicate the specialty, name, address and telephone #.

- Primary Care Physician:

- Dentist:

- Eye Doctor:

- Podiatrist:

- Specialist: (*e.g.,, Oncologist, Urologist, Gynecologist*):

- Specialist:

- Other:

Primary Health Insurance Coverage

Provider:

Policy #:

Contact Person (if any):

Telephone #:

Secondary or Supplemental Insurance

Type of Insurance:

Provider:

Policy #:

Contact Person (if any):

Telephone #:

Other Insurance (e.g., Long-Term Care)

Type of Insurance:

Provider:

Policy #:

Agent's Name:

Telephone #:

Location of Original Policy:

Life Insurance:

Type (*e.g., Term, Variable, etc.*):

Insurance Company:

Policy #:

Agent's Name:

Telephone #:

Location of Original Policy:

Religious Affiliation:

Place of Worship:

Contact Name:

Address:
Telephone #:
Pharmacy (Retail):
Address:
Telephone #:
Contact Person (*if any*):
Pharmacy (Other):
Address:
Telephone #:
Contact Person (*if any*):
Name of Financial Advisor:
Name of Firm:
Telephone #:
Name of Stock Broker:
Name of Firm:
Telephone #:
Primary Financial Institution:
Branch Address:
Type of Account(s):
Account Number(s):

Contact Name:

Telephone #:

Secondary Financial Institution:

Branch Address:

Type of Account(s):

Account Number(s):

Contact Name:

Telephone #:

Location of Safety Deposit Box:

Safety Deposit Box Number:

Location of Safety Deposit Box Key:

Authorized Signatures:

Mortgage Company or Landlord:

Address:

Telephone #:

Acct./Policy #:

Name of Attorney:

Name of Firm:

Telephone #:

Location of Advance Directives:

Location of Will: Person(s) Appointed Power of Attorney:
Driver's License #: State of Issue: Expiration Date:
Summary of Military Service: Location Military Service Records: Honors: Location of Discharge Papers, etc.:
Location of Recent Tax Returns: Tax Specialist: Telephone #:
Credit Card Companies: Account Holders Name (*on each card*): Telephone #: NOTE: Do not List Credit Card #'s.
Detail on in-force Service Contracts: (e.g., alarm monitoring, pest control, lawn service, etc.)

Detail on a pre-arranged or pre-paid Funeral Plans:

Location of written plans or contract:

Funeral Provider:

Contact Name:

Address:

Telephone #:

Location of Cemetery Plots:

Insurance Carriers for Auto, Home, Property & Casualty:

Company Name(s):

Telephone #'s:

Other:

Location of Vehicle Titles:

Location of Deed to House or other Real Estate:

This is not an exhaustive list. Add other information as your situation merits.

"When you look at your life, the greatest happiness es are family happinesses."
– Joyce Brothers

5.

Practical and Purposeful Caregiving

Things are rarely as simple or clear cut as they seem. That is certainly the case of people involved in the care process. As people live longer, there also comes a need to care for those who cannot manage alone. A recent article in the AARP Bulletin entitled *Old, infirmed turn to children*, indicated that there are over 22 million households where family members are caring for aging loved ones, more than third the number of a decade ago. The article stated: *"The growing number reverberates through marriages, savings accounts and workplaces as people try to manage their parents' lives without losing control of their own."* [104] The article also said that while medical breakthroughs allow people to live longer, the quality of life is not always better.

According to the Administration on Aging, older women outnumber older men 21.6 million to 15.7 million. [105] With women living an average of four to five years longer than men, I believe it is important to give consideration to your loved one's skills and abilities should either parent suddenly find him or herself alone. Of the 30 percent of non-institutionalized (a.k.a. community dwelling) older persons who live alone, an estimated 7.8 million are women and 2.9 million are men. And, for women aged 65 and older, 48% live alone.[106] My point in mentioning this is because should an older person live alone, he or she may not have the confidence, skills or abilities to manage aspects of daily living. For example, when my mom was in the hospital my dad did not know how to cook, do laundry and manage other things around the house. Likewise when my dad was in the hospital, my mom would not have paid the bills, put gas in the car, mow the lawn, etc. While every family is different and generationally diverse, be careful not to assume that older generations share the blended roles of younger generations.

As I mentioned in Chapter 1, I believe it is important for people to realize that either role – caregiver or care receiver – is less than ideal for the simple reason that we would all prefer to be free from disease and living active and independent lifestyles. I would much rather have had my mom bouncing her grandkids on her knee, shopping for Easter dresses and cheering them on at school activities than going to visit her in a locked dementia care unit at a local nursing home. I am pretty sure she would have also preferred the same.

In Chapter 4, I mentioned that I teach a graduate level class on aging and adult development. In one of the first classes, I ask my students, who are usually in their early 20s, to share words that describe older adults, I typically hear the usual derogatory terms such as: forgetful, geezers, blue hairs, old farts, stubborn, slow, boring, senile, closed minded, obstinate and one that I hadn't heard until just recently – chicken skin. Then, when I point out that everything said was negative, and I ask for something positive the words I always get are wise or wisdom. What words would you use to describe older adults and your elderly family members? If the words you come up with are more negative than positive, be extra careful to treat your loved ones in a respectful and kind manner.

At a recent class (spring 2009), I mentioned that I find myself acting like my mom sometimes when I go shopping with my daughters. I used to get so frustrated with my mom when she would not go into a store because, *"The music is too loud."* Now, in my late 40s, I find myself saying the same thing. After I shared one of my frustrations, I asked my students to share a few of theirs. One of the most common responses was, *"Old people are so slow."* Other responses included," *[Grandparents] always tell us the same boring stories"* and *"When we go out to eat, she [Grandma] dribbles her food and invariably chokes on something."*

I then asked, *"Do you think they do those things intentionally?"* The point I am trying to make is that certain things may not be the way we like, but that should not diminish the love, value and respect we show others. Frankly, I believe that many older people may tell the same stories as they desperately want to engage and talk with others. The following are a few comments that I have heard from older adults throughout the past few years. These comments, like the ones in the previous chapter, show that many older adults may have frustrations that are similar to the frustrations we may have as caregivers.

- "My biggest frustration is my slowness. I can sense myself reacting slower, moving slower, and processing things slower." – Kathleen, 73 years old

- "I never imagined it would be so hard to open a jar, read a medicine bottle, get up from a sitting position, or comprehend new information. I never imagined so many people would ignore me and view me as being senile." – Vivian, 69 years old

- "One of my biggest frustrations is it seems that nobody wants to pay attention to the so-called 'old guy.' I commanded troops during my time in the military and was treated with the utmost respect and honor. Now that I'm retired it seems I get treated like a child and my opinion means nothing." – Ray, 72 years old

- "I feel invisible as an older woman." – Evelyn, 66 years old

The Caregiver Perspective

Most caregivers have a genuine desire to help and encourage others in ways that are supportive and kind. A challenge, however, is drawing the line between our hopes and desires for others and their own personal aspirations. Many caregivers become paternalistic and act in ways that suggest they know more about what is best for the care receiver than the receiver may know him or herself. While comments are occasionally made that compare older adults to children, I believe nothing could be farther from the truth. While few would dispute the similarities in the parent/child roles, one major difference that makes analogies of older adults as children misleading and inaccurate is that children are 100% dependent on their parents for all of their needs – food, clothing, shelter, etc. [Older] adults on the other hand, unless that a mind-altering disease such as Alzheimer's or are otherwise deem incompetent, have a personal responsibility and right to make decisions for themselves.

Regardless of whether our natural instinct is to be paternalistic, as the saying goes, all we can do is *"Lead the horse to water, but we cannot make it drink."* In other words, the most we can really do is share information, offer perspectives, and encourage our loved ones to make what we believe are wise and healthy choices. Ultimately, until a person is deemed incompetent, we have no real control. For those of you who may disagree, you might be thinking something like, *"But my parents are making some really bad choices that have tremendous consequences on them and even me."* My response to that is *YES*, they very well may be, and that is their choice.

When I speak at conferences, I often ask the audience how many of them have ever made poor decisions in their lives. In addition to me raising both my hands, every hand in the place goes up. My point is that we have all made regrettable choices, and will likely continue to do so. Regardless of whether our choice is to over-indulge in a favorite desert, avoid exercise, or burn the candle on both ends by overdoing things in life – work, family, etc., we all make poor choices now and then (or even regularly). Frankly that is our prerogative. Overcoming a lifetime of ingrained behaviors can be challenging. Making changes that require us to give up bad habits that bring us a sense of pleasure or satisfaction is extremely challenging for most people. In addition, looking past the here and now and seeing the potential long-term benefits is not easy.

So, does that mean if our loved ones are not receptive to our attempts to provide support and encouragement, we should just give up? *Absolutely not.* Instead, I believe that we should continue in a loving and kind way try to share information, offer perspective and express concern about possible consequences to help them realize what we believe. Also, if they make a comment that we disagree with, I believe that not challenging their misinformed judgment actually reinforces and further ingrains their beliefs. For example, if you fail to disagree when someone says, *"At my age, it won't matter anyway,"* it would seem as though you are silently agreeing. If you disagree, ask a question like, *"What makes you say that?"* You could also say, *"Do you really believe that because I certainly do not."* One question we as caregivers should regularly ask ourselves is are we helping or enabling?

Helping vs. Enabling

Finding the right balance between helping someone and encouraging the person to be self-sufficient can be challenging. The tendency is to want to be compassionate and help make life easier, especially for someone who is aging or ill. The reality is that by doing things for people that they could do themselves, we run the risk of enabling.

"Enabling is anything that stands in the way of or softens the natural consequences of a person's behavior." [107] When we enable, we allow a person to become dependent on us – known as codependency. A person who is codependent is, *"Someone who exhibits too much, and often inappropriate, caring for persons who depend on him or her."* [108] To determine how much of an enabler you are, consider how many of the following characteristics are present in relationships for which you are a caregiver.

- Do you do things for the purpose of avoiding conflict?
- Do the things your loved ones do or say tend to control the way you respond?
- Do you feel pity when loved ones face an undesirable situation?
- Do you make excuses to explain the things you do to help others?
- When you take on responsibility, does it make it possible for others to avoid responsibility?
- Do you take on others' problems so that they can avoid making difficult decisions?
- Do you put up with the behaviors of certain people only because they are family?
- Do you fear saying or doing something that you believe might hurt other people's feelings and damage the relationship?

Enabling often makes challenging situations even worse. In situations where there may be legitimate barriers that necessitate assistance, such as lack of money or an inability to drive, the challenge is often making the choice to acknowledge and address the situation. While the balance between helping and enabling varies from person to person, the reasons why people enable tend to be similar – to avoid conflict. Rather than confronting the situation, enablers go along with a decision even when they know it's not in someone's best interest. Here are a couple things to consider when making choices:

- When a loved one expresses a need, regardless of how trivial it is, do you set boundaries or do you continue to respond to the requests over and over again? Foregoing things that are important to you for the sole purpose of accommodating another person's wishes may become a choice you have to live with for life and a source of constant frustration.

- Does your *helping* ultimately get the person what he or she wants without having to make changes? By avoiding situations, we often find ourselves back in the same situation repeatedly.

As the saying goes, *"If a person is hungry, you have two choices. Buy him a fish or teach him how to fish."* If you buy him a fish today, chances are he will be hungry tomorrow. This is not to suggest that we should force people to do everything for themselves. Instead, this is to suggest that it may not make sense to rescue someone for the sake of rescuing without considering the consequences. Often it is our actions or inactions that set a precedent and lead to expectations, many of which may be unreasonable.

Caregiver TLC

So as a caregiver how do I best help? I believe that caregivers should support, encourage and love the care recipient. While different definitions of caregiving already have been shared, caregiving is really all about the Golden Rule, *"Do unto others as you would have them do unto you."* Since that may seem rather vague, think of it as TLC. When I speak of TLC, most people think of the obvious Tender, Loving Care. Additionally, I like to remind people of the importance of Touch, Listen and Coach.

- TOUCH – When words cannot express your feelings or concerns, the best thing may simply be to put your arm around someone or hold his or her hand. Sometimes just being there is all a person wants or needs.

- LISTEN – I am sure you have heard the saying that people have two ears and only one mouth for a purpose. Let your loved ones express their feelings and fears. Avoid the tendency to jump in, take charge and, "*Fix it.*"

- COACH – It can help for caregivers to offer different perspectives to help a care recipient determine what is in their best interest. Pride often gets in the way of people's choices. People needing care do not want to be a burden on their family and friends. Whether they are having trouble maneuvering the steps, occasionally wet themselves or anything else, it is important to reassure them that, "*It's okay,*" while coaching him or her so that future situations or struggles can be avoided.

In regard to how best to help, make sure you have reasonable expectations for yourself and other people that are involved. Do not expect too much, too quickly. Celebrate each small success. Realize that often, the more people try to help, the more they are rejected and criticized. For care recipients, rejection may be a coping mechanism that often serves to create attention or to cover anxiety about being dependent or the perception of being a burden. For some people, negative attention through conflict can be better than no attention at all. Also, do not try to force your opinion on someone else. Make your point and convey why you are suggesting what you are suggesting.

If you want to help, but a loved one rejects your offers, you might help anyway. For example, my dad would reject my offers to do most everything. *"Can I drive you to your doctor's appointment?"* And he would say *"No thanks."* OR *"Can I bring dinner over tonight?* His reply, *"Not necessary."* So what did I do? I did it anyway and found that he really wanted the support; he just did not want to be a burden and was finding it difficult to accept the fact that his life was becoming increasingly challenging. This is not to suggest that all caregivers show *do it anyway.* You will need to determine what is best for your situation knowing your parents.

I have come to realize that many older adults who have been self-sufficient for most of their lives may not know how to accept assistance. While a person may express that no help is necessary, once they start to receive assistance, there is a good chance that the little bit of extra help can be quite nice. In all my years, I have never heard of a person who received a meal from someone who defiantly threw the meal away saying to him or herself, *"I told them I did not want to eat!"*

There can be a fine line between helping too much and not enough. Ideally, family members should think about how they can encourage loved ones. Develop and implement a plan that meets the physical, social and psychological needs of the care recipient. You may also need to help financially. The two types of care plans are: habilitative and rehabilitative.

- Habilitative care, doing more over time, is appropriate in situations where a person is expected to gradually lose the ability to provide self-care and live independently. Since a person's dependence is expected to increase over time, the goal of a habilitative care plan is to help the person to function at their highest possible level.

- Rehabilitative care, doing less over time, is appropriate in situations where a person is expected to make a full or partial recovery. Since a person's dependence is expected to be temporary, the focus of a rehabilitative care plan is to assist and encourage people to relearn or regain skills with the goal of restoring independence.

Besides wanting loved ones to maintain their skills and abilities, I encourage you and your family to place dignity at the top of the list. The concepts behind dignity are twofold – internal and external.

First, it is critical for your loved one to feel important and to have an internal feeling of love and worth. Importance suggests that the care recipient matters, and that he or she has the right to make decisions for him or herself. It does not matter how honorable the intentions of family members and friends might be. As long as the care recipient is competent to make decisions, I believe that he or she should have the final say – whether you agree or disagree.

Second is the concept of respectability or external appearance. Respectability has to do with the presentation of a person – how he or she outwardly appears to others (e.g., appearance, smell). External dignity issues include such things as:

- Incontinence – inability to control one's bladder and bowels
- Mobility – getting around (e.g., walking, cane, wheelchair, etc)
- Dental care – brushing teeth and caring for dentures
- Eye glasses – keeping the lenses clean and prescriptions up-to-date
- Grooming – washing hair, brushing hair, shaving
- Appearance and cleanliness of clothing

Having talked to hundreds and hundreds of people over the years, I have found that care recipients simply want to look respectable, feel valued and not be forgotten.

Person vs. The Circumstances

Let's face it. When a loved one faces a challenge or is labeled with a medical condition, family and friends have a tendency to treat the person differently. I suggest that you treat the person the same as before a medical condition existed. Instead, what you should treat differently is the circumstances. Let me say that again, do not treat the person differently, treat the circumstances differently. When I talk about the circumstances, I am focusing on the environment as opposed to the person.

To demonstrate what I mean, let's assume that a person has a broken leg. If you go over to a friend's house and see that he or she has a broken leg, a natural reaction is to ask what happened and to accommodate the person. Then, over time, you are going to ask how the person is recovering, when he or she is going to get the cast off, how you can be helpful, etc. With illness and disease, many people do not do that. *"The white elephant in the room"* refers to a situation where something is apparent, yet no one is willing to acknowledge it. While not everyone is going to want to talk about their medical concerns, avoiding the issue can create discomfort and anxiety for everyone involved.

If a person has dementia, do not stop loving the person. While the relationship will change over time, the person with dementia will always have a need for connectedness and human touch. To treat the circumstances differently, you may want to take steps to try and reduce potential anxiety, agitation or confusion. For example, try to avoid over-stimulating your loved one or putting them on the spot by asking a complex question.

If a person is experiencing hearing loss, treat him or her with the same loving kindness as before. To address the circumstance of hearing loss, you might reduce background noises, speak slower and louder, and enunciate your words more clearly.

Remember that people want to be defined by their personality, not by a disease. Some people are embarrassed about a condition. Others may be afraid that friends and family will start talking behind their back and treating them differently, often inappropriately.

Heart And Hand Issues

As suggested earlier, TLC issues are centered mainly on the heart and feelings. Hand issues, which are often easier for people to grasp, are more task-oriented.

It is not uncommon for older people to need some assistance with basic tasks. A person who is ill or injured may also have physical needs. Needs are often referred to as daily living activities. As the name suggests daily living activities are those things which a person engages in on a daily basis. These activities are basic to caring for one's self and maintaining independence. Activities are classified into two distinct areas: Activities of daily living (ADLs) and Instrument activities of daily living (IADLs). Although both are critically important, there is a tendency for people to focus on the aspects of personal care.

- ADLs are daily *personal care* activities such as bathing (sponge, bath or shower), getting dressed, getting in or out of bed or a chair (also called transferring), using the toilet, eating, and getting around or walking.

- IADLs are activities about *independent living* and include preparing meals, managing money (writing checks, paying bills), shopping for groceries or personal items, maintaining a residence/performing housework (e.g., laundry, cleaning), taking medications, using a telephone, handling mail, taking care of a pet, and traveling via way of car or public transportation.

Physical or mental limitations may restrict people's ability to perform activities of daily living. When people have a limitation, they have an inability to independently perform one or more daily living activities. A three-part scale is often used to determine dependence or deficit for each activity.

Independent → Assistance Needed → Dependent

- INDEPENDENT suggests a person can perform tasks without assistance.

- ASSISTANCE NEEDED suggests a person can perform tasks with assistance from a human being, support device or both.

- DEPENDENT suggests a person is unable to perform tasks on his or her own.

Why is it important to be aware of a person's limitations with ADLs?

- Recognizing a person's limitations is the first step to developing a care plan to provide the appropriate type and level of assistance.

- Determining the necessary type of ADL care enables families to assign caregiver roles and become educated on how to perform ADL care properly to meet the unique needs of a loved one.

- Admission policies for Adult Day services, care communities and institutions often reflect ADLs to determine eligibility and placement for a certain type of care.

- Long-term care insurance policies often rely on ADL measures (the inability to perform certain ADLs) to determine whether an individual qualifies for benefits.

Avoid The "Let Me Do That" Mentality

When a person faces a limitation, regardless of whether the situation is a result of age, illness or injury, a natural tendency for family and friends is to overcompensate for the person. Someone faces some sort of limitation and people jump in offering to do it for them... *"Let me do that."* Although your gestures may seem like the right thing to do, they are often unnecessary and even demoralizing.

One frequently asked question I receive is, *"Why do you think so many older people resist assistance from family members?"* Many people think the answer is that older people can be stubborn or set in their ways. I have a different philosophy. My guess is that people are hesitant to place themselves in a situation where they become vulnerable. For example, if a loved one accepts a family member's assistance with one activity, how is he going to be able to say no the next time a son or daughter offers to help? In other words, I would rather not accept any help, as opposed to having someone come in, take over and start doing things his or way.

Also, just because you can do something faster does not mean you should, unless the task could be hazardous for your loved one. For example, you might be able to go the mailbox and back in less than a minute. The same task of getting the mail may take a loved one 10-15 minutes. So what? You see, to you it may be only a task – getting the mail. However, to your loved one, it may be an experience. Going outside, hearing the birds chirp, smelling the spring flowers or the fall leaves, or feeling rain drops or the sun on their face. That could be the highlight of someone's day.

Turning Intentions Into Action

All too often when friends are facing a difficult time in life, a natural response might be saying *"I'm always here for you."* Or *"I'm happy to help any way I can."* Comments like these tend not to be effective because the burden of following up is on the person we want to help. People are often reluctant to ask for help as they do not want to be a bother. Just as older adults do not want to be a burden on others, the same goes for caregivers. Just because an older family member does not ask for assistance does not mean he or she does not want or need help. Do not wait for an invitation; instead put your words into action. Also, when your friends ask how they can help you, make a note of it and follow-up within a week or two to see if the person is really serious and if you can count on him or her.

So what kind of help do you or your loved one(s) need? People facing any type of life-changing or life-threatening health issue tend to need three types of support: emotional, informational and instrumental. Also, depending on a person's religious beliefs and practices, spiritual support may also be desired.

Emotional support is more about being than doing. It is relational. You can help by:

- Visiting someone, talking on the phone and sending cards and flowers.

- Participating in social events, such as going shopping, out for dinner, or to the movies.

- Being available to listen, watch TV, play cards, hold someone's hand, and other expressions of friendship and companionship.

- Asking someone questions that show you care. Often when we ask, *"How are you?"* the only answer we want is, *"I'm fine."* Many people will not open up and share what is on their mind and heart until they believe you really care.

Informational support has to do with helping people become aware and gain knowledge that may be helpful now or in the future. You can be supportive by:

- Letting people know of resources you have found to be helpful (e.g., Web sites, books).

- Connecting your loved ones with others you know who have faced a similar situation. People with a similar disease are "experts" in their own hopes, feelings and concerns.

- Encouraging people to participate in a support group. Having an opportunity to connect with others who understand can often be encouraging.

- Inquiring if you can help someone process information he or she may already have. Likewise, you might also offer to be a sounding board for a person to bounce ideas off of.

Instrumental support involves hands-on assistance with activities of daily living (ADLs). Some ways you can provide tangible assistance include:

- Helping with grocery shopping and meals. You might even coordinate a meal plan.

- Providing a ride to a doctor's appointment, running errands or dropping off and picking up kids from school and other activities.

- Assisting with house chores such as taking out the garbage, running the sweeper, doing the dishes, doing the laundry, cutting the grass, pulling weeds, planting flowers, cleaning the gutters, etc..
- Arranging appointments and scheduling services.
- Organizing someone's mail and helping with bill payment activities.

Spiritual support involves providing encouragement and prayer that addresses a person's spiritual needs and religious beliefs. Some ways you can provide spiritual support includes:

- Offering daily prayer, and when together with the person, asking about specific prayer requests.
- Sharing a devotional, scripture or playing comforting music.
- Reflecting on the person's beliefs. Often religious symbols (e.g., a cross on a wall) or the visible presence of a Bible can be an indicator of one's religious beliefs.

Are there others ways you might be supportive to someone who is aging or ill?

Coping Mechanisms

Coping can be especially difficult for families dealing with a chronic illness. In her book *Meeting the Challenge: Living with Chronic Illness*, author and medical psychotherapist Audrey Kron offers some practical advice. She suggests people try to live their lives as normally as possible, be prepared, and pour their feeling out into a creative outlet. I believe her suggestions are appropriate for both caregivers and care receivers.[109]

Do not think solely about your loved one; also consider your needs and feelings. An unhealthy caregiver is of no value to a care recipient. Caregiving is sure to take an emotional toll on you. To help validate yourself, and recognize that you are not alone, you might find it helpful to participate in a support group, at least once in a while. Do not internalize everything and let things get bottled up inside of you. Identify resources and support groups in your area. You will quickly find that most people are ready and eager to help you. To locate support groups in your area, ask a local senior agency or refer to the Health and Wellness section featured weekly in many local newspapers. Also, seek moral support from family and friends. Talk about the emotions you are experiencing, and get things off your chest when you feel burdened.

An example that is often used to demonstrate the importance of the caregiver taking care of oneself is from the airline industry. When the flight attendant is explaining the safety procedures, he or she says, *"In the event a cabin depressurization, air masks will automatically fall from above. If this happens, place your own mask securely around your head before tending to those around you."* The point is that caregivers must make their own health and wellbeing a priority. Take care so you can give care.

A Closing Thought

Do the best you can do, be attentive to the needs of the person for whom you are caring and do not assume you will be told all that is expected of you. In addition to helping with tasks, make sure not to overlook the importance of relationship. Care receivers often value the presence of the adult children, other family members and friends more than we will ever know. In addition, do not beat yourself up if the care needed is beyond what you can personally provide. You will likely wonder if anyone can provide the same loving care as you. After all, you have years and years of experience with your parents, now along comes someone that does not know their feelings, likes, dislikes, etc. One suggestion I have for families who benefit from the help of professional caregivers is to share a bit of life history about the care receiver. You may even wish to share a few photos. Just as the *Look Closer, See Me* poem in Chapter 4 chronicled the lady's life, sharing a few highlights can provide valuable insight and often leads to engaging conversations.

As a caregiver, also be sensitive to your thoughts and feelings. I have vivid memories about my sadness when it became necessary for mom to move into a residential community that specialized in dementia care. While we tried having mom live with us in our home, the stimulation of younger children, pets and constant activity was more than she could cope with. Even though we stand by our decision and believe it was best for her, my sister and I had quite a difficult time dealing with the fact that mom would now be living in a 400-square-foot room in a rather sterile environment. Our frustration was our belief that our mom deserved more. Having lived in a nice, middle-class home all her life, we found it tremendously difficult to see her having to leave the majority of her possessions behind. Basically, she was able to have a bed, chair, table and a few pictures. I guess we all hold out the hope that our parents so called golden years will in fact be golden. Therefore, when disease and functional limitations present challenges, do the best you can do and make sure your motives are honorable. In addition, try to be brave and positive for them, even when it is difficult.

KEY LEARNINGS – *Top three findings from this chapter:*

1.

2.

3.

ACTION ITEMS - *Things you want to do or do differently:*

Check when Completed	*Action Item*	*Target Completion Date*

"When people talk, listen completely.
Most people never listen."
– Ernest Hemingway

6.

Discussions, Decisions and Dynamics

Is it just me, or would you agree that communication is not what it used to be? It seems like with every step forward in technology, the art of conversation takes one step back. I vividly remember the days of sitting in the kitchen or living room with family talking, playing games and spending time together. Granted, those were the days when there were only a handful of television channels, going to a baseball game was a major family outing, and getting an ice cream was a special treat.

Fast-forward to 2010, and technological advances have changed the world. Now a conversation competes with an iPod, channel surfing hundreds of television stations, text messaging, e-mail, Facebook, Twitter and more. When people do engage in two-way communication, the topic of conversation seems to focus on news, weather and sports with life issues often being overlooked or avoided.

Delving into matters that are personal and private can be met with resistance, especially if such conversations are uncomfortable or out of character. I have begun the chapter this way to illustrate that many of us find it beneficial to be more purposeful and personal in our conversations. Equally important is to ensure that what is being communicated is what is being understood. Out of the 2,000 words that are commonly used in daily conversation, *"500 of the words most frequently used have more than 14,000 definitions."* [110] Therefore, it may be helpful to validate that the thoughts you express are, in fact, interpreted and understood the way you intended.

Does the following statement reflect your thoughts about your efforts to communicate?

"I know you believe you understand what you think I said but I am not sure you realize what you heard is not what I meant."

While communication can be hard in everyday life, it can be even more difficult when talking with a loved one who is facing a health-related challenge or is frustrated with, or fearful about, aspects of life. In fact, many families feel uncomfortable talking about perceived problems or don't know how to help or what to do and say. My hope is that these next two chapters provide you with the tips and tools needed to make the most of your conversations.

Respect In Communications

Even though most caregivers have good intentions, the care process can be challenging and good intentions are not always recognized. Remember, it is usually easier for people to give than to receive. Many older adults have been self-sufficient all their lives and find it hard to accept support. Stress behaviors, including arguing and resistance, tend to emerge when people face challenging or unexpected situations.

Many older adults are facing a range of emotions, and it can be difficult for younger, able-bodied people to grasp what their life is like. In October 2009, we conducted a simulation exercise at the University of Cincinnati College of Nursing with a group of industrial design students. Designing solutions for health care, as part of a collaborative effort with the College of Design, Architecture, Art, and Planning (DAAP), we felt it was important that the students experience life from the perspective of a hospital patient. Sometimes the best way to learn and understand something is to experience it. The students quickly realized that people often respond uncharacteristically when facing challenges and frustrations. The following two stories illustrate situations that can have an adverse effect on a person's quality of life.

In one of our simulations, a student was in a hospital bed with one of her arms restricted. When it was time to eat her meal, she responded, *"I don't think I'm that hungry."* In fact, she was hungry, but she found it so difficult to eat that it was easier to skip the meal, an uncharacteristic response.

When asked about her patient experience afterward, she said, *"Even in the short amount of time, the feelings of helplessness is very acute. Needing help with easy things like moving the tray and having to depend on other people is frustrating. You look for things and ways you can do stuff on your own. When people tried to help me with stuff I could do on my own I found myself resenting them. People want to be capable."*

Another student playing the role of a patient wore glasses that made it difficult to see clearly, and had cotton in his ears to simulate hearing loss. He was quite antsy being alone so he got out of bed to go find someone — anyone. When asked about his experience, he said, *"Walking around is not fun, nor is sitting here. Since I can't see anything, I'm just kind of stuck here. I feel frustrated because I can't do anything on my own. I feel inadequate."*

If you or a loved one felt frustrated or inadequate, can you image how you might react with actions and words? Our behaviors often reflect our emotions to a particular circumstance. So, just as the one student opted not to eat, imagine how loved ones may choose to struggle through life, rather than putting themselves in a vulnerable position or risk burdening others.

Understand that talking with loved ones about their personal matters and affairs can be awkward for everyone involved. Try to sympathize with your loved one's thoughts and feelings. This requires talking to loved ones in a respectful manner, hearing concerns, understanding values, and finding ways to provide the support they need and want. Respectful communication also avoids belittling them by using terms that are can be viewed as condescending. Patronizing a loved one can cause emotional pain and suffering. [111] Avoid it all costs.

The following is a passage from Rev. Eric H.F. Law's *Respectful Communication Guidelines:*

"**R** – Take responsibility for what you say and feel without blaming others (Use "I" statements, not "you").

E – Empathetic listening.

S – Be sensitive to differences in communication styles.

P – Ponder what you hear and feel before you speak.

E – Examine your own assumptions and perceptions (Why am I reacting/feeling this way?).

C – Confidentiality can uphold the wellbeing of the community.

T – Tolerate ambiguity, because we are not here to debate who is right or wrong." [112]

In terms of the outcome of a conversation, participants are often focused on winning or losing as opposed to understanding each other's point of view. The outcome does not have to be my way, no way, half way, or your way. Instead, be open to what others have to say and why. Also, keep in mind that people are generally more open to discussing their health and care issues when the needs are not imminent. Doing so tends to give people more of a sense of control over important aspects of life.

Identity And Responsibility

In addition to considering both verbal and non-verbal aspects, consider the significance of communication with everyone involved in the care process. Care receivers, whether consciously or subconsciously, are always assessing risk and reward. They are basically weighing the perceived importance of issues, the perceived implications, making a judgment about their situation, skills and abilities, and ultimately choosing whether to address an issue, and if so, to what extent. For example, your loved one may or may not acknowledge a medical diagnosis and/or that daily living activities are becoming more challenging and exhausting.

The more willing and able people are to acknowledge and accept the reality of their situation, the more likely they are to consider options and alternatives. Likewise, if loved ones are in denial or minimize the severity of a situation, they are more likely to be resistant to any sort of change until such time as status quo is no longer feasible.

For years, two of the most purported fears of older adults have been dying and outliving one's assets. However, a recent survey of 800 people indicated, *"Senior citizens fear moving into a nursing home and losing their independence more than they fear death."* [113] The findings from the *Aging in Place in America* study may not be statistically significant, but it highlights an issue many older adults fear – losing their independence.

Independence and identity are often at the heart of concerns and conversations about living arrangements, care needs, driving and more. For example, findings from research about driving indicated, *"Older adults were more likely to place emphasis on the threat that driving reduction or cessation posed to their identity as an independent person than the risk associated with crashing or citations."* [114] Quite often, autonomy concerns affect the communication process and make options favoring independence more attractive regardless of how *at risk* a care receiver may be. Likewise, people who fear losing their independence may resist support and change in order to avoid feeling frail, sick, compromised or old.

In addition to the care receiver's thoughts and feelings, the caregiver often feels a tremendous responsibility to ensure their loved ones' safety and wellbeing. Family members often feel compelled to initiate conversations, encourage changes, and establish restrictions that may conflict with the care receiver's need for independence and control. In some cases, adult children may even try to reach a consensus with others without the knowledge of or input from the care recipient.

While health care and social services professionals may provide valuable insight and direction, be careful not to ambush an older adult and force a solution you perceive to be ideal. Doing so can be demoralizing and is typically unnecessary.

Even though the intentions of family and friends may be honorable, a natural response for many people is to step in and take over when a loved one faces illness, injury or age-related functional challenges. Before strapping on a Superman cape and coming to the loved one's rescue, it is important to explore and understand the concept of autonomy and recognize that individuals have the right to their own beliefs and values. The exception may be unsafe or hazardous driving where a loved one may risk personal injury and/or injury or death to others.

Self-determination is a right that can be especially important to people facing any type of age- or health-related loss. Regardless of age, adults have the right to choose how they live their lives as long as they are of sound mind and not subjecting themselves, or others, to harm through self-neglect.

Self-neglect refers to situations where an older adult becomes unwilling or unable to care for him or herself and whose behaviors threaten his or her own health or safety. Many families struggle to determine when a loved one can no longer cope and it is time to step in; however, it will often become apparent. When a person is unwilling or unable to provide for him or herself, the indicators include:

- A person's personal care behaviors cause concern about hygiene, infection and overall health.

- A person is unable to manage his/her medication regimen, which leads to health problems.

- The home often becomes cluttered with junk and laundry. The house becomes dirty, presenting both safety and health concerns.

- A change in eating habits often becomes apparent through sudden weight loss or a decline in overall wellbeing. The cupboards and refrigerator are often bare or contain expired foods.

If you have concerns, but are not sure your loved one needs assistance, trust your instincts. People with moderate or mid-stage Alzheimer's disease or dementia often require assistance due to major gaps in memory and deficits in cognitive function such as decision-making. Also, do not ignore actions and behaviors which you believe are problematic. All too often caregivers would prefer to avoid the white elephant in the room than talk about legitimate issues and concerns. I personally believe that if a caregiver does not acknowledge and voice concerns when an older adult's actions and behaviors seem unsafe or out of character, he or she essentially affirms the care receiver's conduct and indicates acceptance.

Gathering Information

Communication is vital because in order for a care receiver's wishes to be carried out, they must be made known. The challenge is that they do not have a clear understanding of what their loved ones value and want, therefore they are more likely to impose their own preferences. If you are, or anticipate becoming, a caregiver but have not spoken to your loved one about their wishes, it may be time for you to start asking a few questions. There is a high probability you will be called upon at some point to provide assistance.

I suggest caregivers start by asking questions and observing their loved ones in a variety of situations throughout the day and night. The more information you gather, the more likely you will understand and honor their challenges, fears, frustrations, preferences and values. If you make random assumptions and opinionated statements, the more likely you are to face controversy and experience a breakdown in communication.

When talking with family members about ideas or concerns, you may find it beneficial to use *"I"* statements rather than *"You"* statements. *I* statements are less threatening and often better received. In addition, be careful about making opinionated statements as they have a tendency to come across as negative and undermining if others have different opinions.

For example, if you say something like, *"I think you are unsafe to live at home and should move to a nursing home"* or, *"It makes no sense to me that at your age you are still driving"* the person to whom those statements are directed is likely to become defensive. On the other hand, questions have a tendency to suggest a desire to understand, an openness to discuss and a willingness to work together. For example, *"How safe do you feel driving based on your health and all the medications you're taking?* Or, *"Based on your concerns about daily living and keeping up with the house, what can we do to support you and help you get the services you need?"*

If you have not already broached conversation to understand your loved one's wishes and preferences, I highly recommend doing so before you find yourself facing a crisis situation. When you ask questions, do not be discouraged if your loved ones are not forthcoming with answers. Just because you ask a question does not mean they will respond. Often it takes time to build trust and demonstrate true caring before loved ones will open up.

For example, at some point it will be important to understand your loved one's financial situation and his or her ability to meet living and associated care expenses; however, it could be perceived as being selfish and overly concerned with inheritance. Likewise, if a loved one is inadequately prepared for retirement or is facing the misfortune of investments that soured, he or she may wish to avoid discussions and possible embarrassment.

The following are a few questions you may wish to ask. I am not suggesting you ask the questions in the order they appear or word for word as I have written them. Instead, use your own words and ask the questions you think are most important given your situation. Do not overwhelm your loved one — limit the number of questions you ask to two or three at a time.

1. How is aging consistent with or different than *you* expected?

2. Are there any medical conditions that *you* are currently facing or hereditarily predisposed to that might be an indicator of future health-related challenges?

3. As a result of *your* (insert diagnosis), are there certain aspects of life *you* are finding to be more difficult that we can proactively address?

4. If something ever happens to *you*, what would *you* want me (or us, as a family) to do?

5. What are the roles and expectations *you* have for family members in terms of providing assistance, support, etc.?

6. If we are concerned about *your* safety, how can we effectively express our concerns? What would *you* want us to do?

7. Have *you* planned, or otherwise given consideration, for long-term care and LTC insurance?

8. If *you* require assistance with daily living activities or personal care, how would *you* like that provided?

9. If *you* need assistance at some point, do *you* have a preference in terms of where *you* would like to live and how *you* would like us to help you meet your care needs?

10. What type of care/living arrangements are the least desirable to *you* and why?

11. Have *you* executed legal documents including a Will, Power of Attorney, Living Will and Power of Attorney for Health Care?

    a. If YES, where are copies of the documents located? Where is the original Will located? Who is appointed to make decisions for *you* should you be unable? What are *your* preferences about CPR? Would *you* want to be resuscitated or would *you* prefer to allow a natural death?

b. If NO, encourage your parent or loved one to execute the basic documents.

12. Are there certain personal possessions that *you* want to go to specific people?

13. Have you planned for *your* retirement and saved money to cover your typical expenses? What type of assumptions have *you* factored into your retirement plan in regards to living and care expenses? For example, how many years do *you* assume your money will need to last? What is *your* projected life expectancy? What are *your* expectations for personal expenses?

14. What types of assets are at *your* disposal should *you* need funds to cover any sort of medical or care expenses (e.g., cash value in life insurance, long-term care insurance, equity in a house)?

15. What type of health insurance do *you* have, and do *you* expect it to be sufficient for the future?

16. If *you* should become unable to care for yourself or die, what would *your* wishes be for (insert name of spouse)? Do *you* have concerns *you* would like the family to be aware of?

Understanding And Navigating Personalities

As I am sure you know, personality types and family dynamics affect the decision-making process. While there are many different exercises to help people decipher personality types, one of the best known and most respected is the Myers-Briggs Type Indicator (www.myersbriggs.org). I mention Myers-Briggs is because one way to enhance conversation is to speak with people in a way that recognizes their personality characteristics and factors in how they are most likely to participate.

In terms of personality types, know that no one is good, bad, better or worse than another. While personality characteristics can be different, even polar opposites, each is useful and important. To help identify and understand differences, the following is a brief look at the types.

Extraversion (E)/Introversion (I) has to do with how people are energized.

- Extraverts are action-oriented, spontaneous thinkers who process their thoughts by talking aloud. They enjoy interaction with others. Their motto is Ready, Fire, Aim. Extraverts are likely to tell you what they are thinking — you just need to listen.

- Introverts can be sociable, but they have a need for peace and quiet to concentrate, reflect, understand and recharge their batteries. Their motto is Ready, Aim, Aim. Introverts are less likely to be forthcoming with their thoughts and opinions. Therefore, you may need to ask an introvert what he/she is thinking, and then stop talking.

Sensing (S)/Intuition (I) reflects how people take in information.

- Sensors are detail-oriented and tend to rely on their five senses. They want to know the facts. Sensors can be so methodical that decisions are delayed.

- Intuitives rely more on their imagination and what can be seen in *"the mind's eye."* They tend to look for the big picture and seek out patterns and relationships. Intuitives rely more on their hunches. They may have their heads in the clouds and need to be grounded.

Thinking (T)/Feeling (F) refers to how people make decisions.

- Thinkers tend to make decisions based on logic, principle and objective criteria. Thinkers tend to be impersonal, analytical, and need to realize that feelings are facts that need to be taken into consideration when making decisions.

- Feelers focus on a person's needs and values as they make decisions. They are the ones who try to ease differences and seek common ground. Feelers are more personal, seek harmony, and need to realize that even though thinkers' feelings may not be as pronounced or obvious, they also have feelings.

Judging (J)/Perceptive (P) has to do with people's attitudes to the outside world.

- Judging types tend to be decisive, action-oriented, focused on completing tasks, and meeting deadlines. Judgers are regimented planners. Conversations that do not advance the plan or address the desired outcome can be frustrating.

- Perceptive types are more likely to explore options, postpone action and express curiosity. Preceptors are more spontaneous and adaptable. They start many tasks and often find it difficult to complete tasks regardless of a deadline.

While Myers-Briggs is a comprehensive form of evaluation, it may be helpful to jot down what you believe are your tendencies and the tendencies of others involved in the care process. For example, my wife is an ISFP, whereas I am an EITJ. You may also want to complete the personality assessment to better understand factors that can enhance family dynamics. Being aware of and sensitive to personality types can be fun, demonstrate a willingness to enhance communication and have reasonable expectations of each other, and help people communicate more effectively.

The Birds And The Bees Analogy

Many people do not want to talk about aging and long-term care because it may conjure a fear of losing independence or be viewed as an invasion of privacy. I equate the talk Baby Boomers need to have with their aging parents with the talk that our parents had with us years ago about the birds and the bees. I think the analogy of the two talks is quite relevant for a couple of reasons.

1. The talk is not intended to be easy and spur of the moment. It is something that people should prepare for, take seriously and realize that loved ones may soon enter a new stage in life, if they have not already.

2. The first few words can make or break it. Just as you may have rolled your eyes or felt uncomfortable, your loved one may find talking about such serious issues difficult. Chances are, you will either get their attention and there will be a mutual appreciation for having a conversation, or the barriers go up and not much will be accomplished.

The point of the talk is ultimately to understand your loved one's wishes and expectations. If your attempt at meaningful conversation is redirected, or becomes uncomfortable or hostile, you might suggest a few reasons for wanting to have the conversation, such as:

- To ensure loved ones have given consideration to and completed some sort of health care and estate planning.

- To understand and be able to carry out loved ones' wishes should they become incapable of making their own decisions.

Who Should Participate?

One thing to consider is who should participate in family conversations/meetings? There are no right or wrong answers. Depending on the intended topic of conversation, certain people may or may not be included. For example:

- Talks may take place between family members and will not include the current or potential care recipient. For example, adult children can get together to discuss when to have the initial conversation, who might be most appropriate to initiate the idea of having a talk, and what to cover in an initial discussion.

- Certain topics of conversation, such as financial matters may be limited to the immediate family.

- Conversations having to do with a loved one's day-to-day care might include those people who are likely to be actively involved in the care process.

- If certain family members live out of town, you might need to make decisions about moving forward with or without a particular family member(s) or plan conversations during a holiday or another family gathering.

Regardless of who is involved in the conversations, it may be helpful to develop an agenda, formally or informally, so participants know what to expect and have time to prepare. In addition, an agenda can help focus the conversation and keep people from going off on tangents. An agenda might include the following topics and flow:

1. Current Situation — What is the latest on a care receiver's medical diagnosis and prognosis? Are there certain changes or events that merit discussion or review?

2. Feelings Check — How is everyone feeling? For example, are you overwhelmed, scared, angry, etc.

3. Needs — What needs to be accomplished or done differently? Why? Is everyone in agreement? Why or why not? What is the goal or desired outcome from the conversation? Are there certain healthcare, financial or legal concerns that need to be addressed? Is one caregiver asking other family members to share in the care?

4. Roles and Responsibilities — Who wants to do what? What specific limitations do people have in regards to time or location that need to be recognized? Who is going to do what in terms of making decisions, coordinating care, handling personal affairs and interacting with the medical team? Also, how often is each family member planning to contact a parent by telephone or in person?

5. Agreement — Divide and conquer. Agree how to keep everyone up-to-date. Plan the next meeting.

Conversations can be daunting for the care recipients, so be careful not to overwhelm them with too much at once. Regardless of what you are hoping to accomplish, remember you are dealing with real people who matter and have feelings. While it can be helpful to try and maintain order, be careful not to come across as rigid and impersonal. Also, make sure everyone has a chance to be heard. If a particular family member is more outspoken, maybe another family member needs to ask him or her to give other people a chance to be heard. Consider the *here and now* and *the future*. Do not waste time looking back and pointing blame.

Depending on the topic and who participates, the purpose of an initial conversation might simply be to gain consensus that there is a need to talk on a consistent basis and that there are real issues that the family will want to address soon.

Engaging A Loved One

Now that you have a handle on the *what* and *who,* it is time to approach and attempt to engage the care recipient(s) and/or your loved ones with whom you wish to support. I find the approach is just as important to consider as the discussion itself. The following are three approaches I find work well. Consider which one might work best for you.

1. Scripted — With the scripted approach, you plan ahead and notify your loved ones that you would like to talk. I believe that advance notice is critical so no one feels ambushed, caught off guard, unprepared or backed into a corner. With this approach, you simply call a loved one and request a get-together. For people that attend my seminars, I suggest that they say something like: *"Hey dad, I just read this great book about caregiving, and I got to thinking that there are a lot of things I don't know that I probably should have a handle on. Can we get together over the weekend and talk? I'd like to ask you some questions and find out your preferences and expectations should anything ever happen to you or mom."* With this approach, both parties have a chance to reflect and prepare. When you arrive for the talk, there should be no surprise when you start asking questions.

2. Spontaneous — Many people seem to have their guard up and may not be interested in sharing or discussing personal matters. When this occurs, look for a situation that may noticeably impact your loved one. For my dad, the situation was the death of one of his best friends. When he learned of his friend's death, many realities appeared to have set in, enabling me to see his softer side. This was my opportunity to tell him that, as a result of his friend's death, *"I now realize that there are many things I don't know about your and mom's wishes should anything ever happen to either of*

you." Then, start asking questions or agree to sit down in a week or so to talk.

3. Lead By Example — Get your own personal affairs in order so you are able to speak from experience. In this case, you might be able to share some of your plans and planning documents. For example, I could have said to my dad, *"I have planned and organized my personal affairs for the benefit of Karen (my wife) and our daughters should anything ever happen to me. Can I talk to you about some of the things I have done to make life easier should I predecease Karen? Also, I would like to talk to you about your wishes should you predecease mom?"* If you are unsure of what, if anything, your loved one has done in terms of planning, you could ask, *"Have you given much consideration to your wishes and what you would like or expect me to do?"*

Regardless of how you initiate the conversation, consider where to hold a discussion so that everyone is comfortable and in an appropriate setting. A private setting, such as a home or office may provide less distractions, whereas a public setting may be preferential as it is a neutral site and no one has 'home field' advantage. Also, if one parent seems reluctant to talk about him or herself, it may be easier to ask about wishes for his or her spouse. Ask dad about mom — what does he want for her should anything happen to him? Removing dad as the topic of conversation, and focusing on mom, can often be an effective.

Have Reasonable Expectations

While conversations can be an effective and essential way get family members on the same page, don't expect miracles to happen overnight. I often use the analogy of planting seeds. In other words, you may introduce a concern today that will not be acted upon for weeks, months or even years to come. If there is not immediate acceptance, change or results, don't give up or feel like you failed. People often need to become aware of something and have time to process the issues and potential consequences before being ready, willing and able to make a choice. Likewise, if something seems obvious to you, yet others do not see things similarly, try expressing yourself differently and sharing what you believe are the risks and rewards, and why. I personally believe that changes occur when the perceived benefits of change outweigh the perceived consequences of status quo.

A Closing Thought

As a caregiver for my parents, I have vivid memories of them being oblivious to issues that were obvious to me. Over the years, I have come to realize so much of my frustration was trying to control things over which I had absolutely no control. Looking back, I realize I wasted a lot of time and energy trying to persuade and pressure my parents to make changes that I thought were best for them. Not only did this strain our relationship, it also got us nowhere. The more effective approach is to understand and honor their wishes and preferences. Instead of trying to force them to move to Assisted Living, I wish I would have been more open to exploring ways to make their home environment work better for them.

Older adults and people facing limitations due to health challenges have a need to maintain control. As people experience more losses (e.g., strength, energy, health, friends) control becomes increasingly important. Sometimes the only way an older person can maintain control is to say, "No." Often confused with stubbornness, caregivers waste precious time trying to show our beloved care recipients the error of their ways.

Do not make the mistake of trying to force your opinion, second-guessing them on important issues, and ultimately stripping them of control. Arguing drains energy. Instead, back off and stop badgering someone to do something. The more we give control, the more likely they are to take responsibility for their lives. For the benefit of the care recipient(s) and the caregiver(s), I suggest that when you and your family focus on an issue, give considerable thought to what you are trying to accomplish and why. Then, focus on the things that matter.

An article entitled *Oh, grow up!* offers the following advice to adult children desiring a healthy, peer relationship with their parents.

- *"Avoid topics and conversations you know are problematic.*

- *Decide what's worth arguing about and what you should ignore.*

- *Acknowledge what your mother says, but don't overreact.*

- *Weigh how much of the annoyance comes from your mother and how much is actually pressure you are putting on yourself.*

- *Bear in mind, it's not important that you always be "right."*

- *Don't be afraid to ruffle your mother's feathers.*

- *Be aware of what you want from your mother and what she is capable and prepared to give."* [115]

KEY LEARNINGS – *Top three findings from this chapter:*
1.
2.
3.

ACTION ITEMS - *Things you want to do or do differently:*		
Check when Completed	*Action Item*	*Target Completion Date*

"Honest disagreement is often
a good sign of progress."
– Mahatma Gandhi

7.

Communication Strategies in Conflict

Open and honest communication between family members is ideal and important; however, it may not always happen or be easy. While the idea of talking with one another may seem simple, it can actually become quite complex when fears, frailty, frustration and family are involved. Misunderstandings occur, tempers flare, and personality types and styles emerge, as do past hurts. Family dysfunction, dynamics and differing agendas are a few of the many factors that can complicate communication.

Another challenge is that care receivers and caregivers are often working from different agendas.

- Care receivers may be concerned about maximizing independence, maintaining control, coping with functional losses and the loss of friends, dying and more.

- Caregivers tend to be more concerned about health and medical issues, living and care arrangements, preparing for the inevitable and their loved ones' coping ability, loneliness and financial wellness.

I know from being a dad how the agendas of parents and children are seldom aligned and the challenges that result. Now add the fact that many of the care receivers' and caregivers' concerns are likely to be about life-changing or life-threatening issues, so there is an even greater potential for conflict.

Each family has a unique history and dynamic that affects interactions. While conflict may make discussion difficult and even uncomfortable, I strongly suggest family members try to work through issues of concern, rather than ignore them. Remember, ignoring an issue does not solve the issue. Also, just because you address something, the outcome may not always be positive. For example, attempts of caregivers to be supportive could be viewed as bulldozing and getting involved in areas they may have no business. Trying to convince a person that his or her functional limitations warrant the need for help could highlight physical or cognitive deficits causing an older person to panic and take potentially inappropriate and extreme measures. Likewise, attempts to help a person manage life during periods of transition could strike fear about change and reinforce his or her inability to cope. Just as there are two sides to every coin, honest attempts to be supportive may not be viewed as such.

As you will quickly discover, if you have not already, patience is a virtue and one that will likely be tried and tested throughout your caregiving experience. I occasionally find that caregivers can be their own worst enemy thinking everything is a crisis. As the *Caregiver Bill of Rights* from Chapter 2 indicated, caregivers do not need to be responsive to every whim and request a loved one has. In fact, responding to issues as though they require immediate attention and resolution can create self-imposed crises when something is not an actual do-or-die situation.

In this chapter, I share a number of suggestions I have found to work quite well. If you find yourself getting nowhere after trying these tactics and using these tools, and you believe that the people and personalities involved make productive conversations impossible, consider engaging the services of a geriatric care manager or a social worker. Unbiased outsiders may be able to facilitate discussions and provide counsel to your family.

Expectations vs. Example

Okay, so we all know there are things we should do for our own health and wellbeing. For example, we should all:

- Drink six to eight 8 oz. glasses of water every day.

- Eat five servings of fruits and vegetables every day.

- Get at least eight hours of sleep every night.

- Engage in vigorous exercise for at least 30 minutes, five times a week.

- Avoid tobacco, excessive use of alcohol and recreational drugs.

- Wear a seatbelt when we are in a moving vehicle.

So how would you rate yourself on these health behaviors? If you are like most people, myself included, chances are you have some room for improvement. The reason I ask about a few of your personal health behaviors is to point out there are certain things we have all heard and likely believe to be wise; however, we do not do them. Why? Is it because we are creatures of habit? Change is hard? The potential consequences of doing what is expected do not seem pertinent? We procrastinate? We just need to get through the current season of our life? We claim it is a New Year's resolution? Or do we pursue healthier behaviors, but give up too quickly because the results are not immediately apparent?

We all have different reasons for making choices, and we will eventually pay the consequences of our choices. For most of us, I believe that until we start to experience the negative consequences and discover the severity of our actions or inactions, maintaining status quo is easiest because the least amount of effort is involved. I used to opt for a more sedentary lifestyle and the convenience of fast food and soda, but when my primary care physician informed me my cholesterol levels and triglycerides count were putting me at an increased risk for a heart attack, that was all I needed to hear. Even though I knew the importance of diet and exercise, and I knew deep down I was making poor choices, it took the fear of having a heart attack to make me suddenly change my behavior.

My reason for mentioning health behaviors and briefly sharing my recent encounter is to demonstrate that having knowledge of what we should do and actually doing those things can be quite different. As a caregiver, you will undoubtedly know and believe there are things that your loved ones should start doing and stop doing. While caregivers often think they know best, intervening or attempting to rescue loved ones from their situation will likely not be well-received and will become a major source of stress. Just as we ourselves have not made certain changes that we know might benefit us, be careful not to unreasonably think your loved ones are going to suddenly embrace change when you express concerns. While this is clearly oversimplified, I find that people approach change in one of the following three ways:

1. Voluntarily make changes. People in this category are proactive, and once they become aware of a concern, they make a personal choice to explore possibilities and make changes. They often sense a change in their skills and ability, and may be uneasy in a current situation.

2. Reluctantly make changes. Over time, these people come to accept that life is becoming increasingly difficult. They try to recognize their limitations, and even though they would prefer life as it is, they know is not realistic and they pursue changes. Family members and friends often play an important role by convincing loved ones that there is a better, easier or safer way. People in this category often need encouragement and prodding when deciding to make significant changes.

3. Resist making any changes. In addition to being extremely stubborn, people in this category often have unrealistic confidence in their situation, skills and abilities. They often express a need to maintain status quo as they feel there are no suitable and satisfactory alternatives, and that may be true. When family or friends express concern, a common response is often *"you just don't understand."* Most older adults have been self-sufficient all their lives and may also have a difficult time depending on, asking for or accepting support from others.

Extreme Situations

The following is an extreme situation that few caregivers will encounter. I share it not to discourage, but rather to point out how complex communication can be, so that you have a general understanding of all that you may be up against.

As a health educator, I enjoy exploring and understanding factors that influence health behaviors. There are numerous models and theories that explain why people behave a certain way and what has to occur before they are ready, willing and able to change behaviors. I find that applying a model is a great way to understand these behaviors, especially when facing immense challenges and extreme situations. For the scenario below, I refer to the PRECEED-PROCEDE Model.[116] The focus is on the first three letters of the word Preceed which stand for **P**redisposing, **E**nabling and **R**einforcing factors.

Situation — The woman's father continues to drive even though he could easily be considered unsafe. On more than one occasion, he has reportedly fallen asleep behind the wheel at a stop sign or stop light. There are numerous scratches and dents on his car. His daughter has expressed concern about his driving multiple times, yet he continues to drive. She does not like confrontation, and she knows how important driving is to her father's identity and independence. He recently ran into a fire hydrant and totaled his car. Fortunately, no one was injured or killed. Unfortunately, he was not cited by the police for any of these incidents. After totaling his car, he went out and bought a new car. It was not long before he hit something and the mirror on the passenger side was left dangling. Not long after that, he plowed over two mailboxes. Again, no one was injured and no citations were issued. While it may seem apparent that this gentleman is unsafe to drive, he has a valid driver's license, he is insured and he owns a car. By applying the *"PRE"* part of the model, you will understand why his daughter's attempts have not achieved the desired outcome — his driving cessation.

Predisposing factors — He has certain knowledge, attitudes and beliefs that lead him to drive, despite his daughter's efforts to get him to stop driving. Unless a crisis occurs that forces him to stop driving, before his behavior changes, his stinking thinking must change. Situations like these often require tough love through which caregivers must challenge their loved ones. While it is unlikely that a single conversation will cause him to stop driving, do not underestimate the value of seeds you are essentially planting. Just as with seeds, cultivating the soil and watering the seeds takes time and effort. After awhile, you hope to see results. Some of the questions the daughter could ask her father that might cause him to change his belief system include:

1. Health — Does her father understand that as he ages, he will naturally encounter certain biological changes (e.g., vision, hearing, strength, reflexes) that are likely to affect his ability to safely operate and control his car? Remember, older adults tend to have an exceedingly positive perception of their state of health; therefore, to what extent is he aware of his medical problems and any functional limitations that result? What does he think about his falling asleep while behind the wheel? Does he think that is normal and okay? Does he realize that the consequences could have been severe? What would he say if he had injured or killed someone?

2. Assessment — Is he willing to take a driver's assessment, including a behind the wheel test? Will he enroll in a driving course (e.g., AARP course, AAA Roadwise Review™) in an effort to sharpen his driving skills? Are there certain medications he is taking for which 'operating machinery' is not advised? Why does he believe his driving is necessary? What alternatives are available so he would not need to drive, and what are his thoughts about each? What is it going to take to get him to stop driving — having his license revoked or killing someone?

3. Performance — What does this gentleman think about his past incidents? Does he realize the severity of the situation? Does he feel comfortable behind the wheel of a car, or does he keep driving because he feels he must? Does he know he has been at fault? Does he understand how fortunate he has been that no one has been injured or killed? Does he think his driving is suddenly going to get better? How would he respond if his daughter had similar incidents? If one of my daughters has a minor incident after she starts driving, we might chalk it up to inexperience; however, if multiple

incidents occur, I would certain intervene. How would he want you to respond?

These and other questions can help you gain an understanding of what he is thinking. They will also help you know what you might need to overcome in order for him to change his thinking and be willingly stop driving. Frequently, people regard driving as a right. However, driving is not a right, it is a privilege, and simply limiting his driving to when conditions may be the safest (e.g., daylight hours, dry road, staying off the highway) might not be enough. Driving is a concern that family and friends may need to address, especially if loved ones are unable or unwilling to make the decision to stop driving. As you discover why he continues to drive, challenge his thinking, share concrete examples and educate him on the severity of the situations, his options and more.

*R*einforcing factors — Regardless of what you discover as you explore the predisposing factors, know that there may be other factors reinforcing his belief that he needs to drive and that he is doing so safely. For example, having a driver's license and insurance coverage may lead him to believe that driving is okay. Likewise, if the police have not cited him for any of the incidents, and they have not intervened, they are essentially suggesting it is okay for him to drive. You could call the local police department, express your concern and ask them for suggestions. If his friends are willing to be passengers in his car, their presence may indicate they trust him. If his son who lives out of state minimizes the severity of his incidents and tells him to *"Be more safe,"* he too is reinforcing his belief that driving is okay.

*E*nabling factors — If he goes to the local Bureau of Motor Vehicles (BMV), and they do not have the heart to tell him they cannot renew his license because he did not pass the driving or vision test, chances are he will be convinced he is okay to drive. If someone reluctantly goes with him to purchase a new car, he will likely interpret his or her presence and participation as an indication that his driving is okay. When his primary care physician or nurse practitioner makes a passing comment that he shouldn't drive at night, he may interpret that to mean certain hours of day. As a result, he may think it is okay to drive in the morning darkness. He may tell his daughter his self-imposed restrictions, such as staying off the highway, avoiding rush-hour traffic and staying home when the roads are slick are safety measures that go above and beyond what is expected of him. Often, when police and medical professionals tell someone they are unsafe to drive and need to stop, the person will listen and respect their authority. Unfortunately, many people in positions of authority do not realize they are enabling a potentially unsafe driver and contributing to his or her risky behavior.

Do you see what you may be up against? Realize that many different people (whether knowingly or subconsciously) have the potential to undermine your efforts to achieve the desired outcome — dad ceasing to drive. People who continue driving even though they are considered unsafe are unlikely to respond to logic or common sense. They may have unrealistic confidence in their driving skills and abilities, or believe they have the right to drive; after all they have had 40, 50 or 60 years experience. As a result, they may keep driving until one of the following occurs:

- They are unable to pass the vision test required to renew their driver's license and the BMV actually fails them.
- Their license is revoked.
- They are denied or do not qualify for auto insurance.
- Injury, illness or deteriorating health makes it unrealistic for a person to drive.
- A vehicle is no longer operational, whether due to an

accident, neglect of maintenance, or the car being disabled.

Note: While I indicated earlier in the book that I whole-heartedly believe older adults have the right to make their own decisions as long as they are of sound mind, this driving scenario is one where the family may need to intervene for the safety of their dad, other drivers and pedestrians. Even though the individuals mind appears sound, in this situation, the physical changes and challenges increase the potential for unsafe driving. One of the most difficult choices family members have to make is whether or not to intervene when there are obvious safety risks. There is a risk in not intervening when you know a person is putting him or herself and others at risk. If something does happen, you must live with the knowledge that it could have been avoided. Reflect on that thought. For more information about Driving, refer to my book entitled *Engaging While AGING*.

Empathy vs. Sympathy

Related to enabling is the need to distinguish between empathy and sympathy. This will help you understand effective ways to support and communicate with elderly loved ones who find themselves at a crossroads. While the dictionary defines them similarly, they are quite different.

Have you ever made a comment like, *"Until they walk a mile in my shoes, they'll never understand?"* Empathy is what we do to try to understand another person's situation and feelings. For example, a sympathy comment like *"I completely understand how you must feel,"* would come across as inappropriate unless you have personally experienced a situation that is almost identical to what the other person is going through.

Sympathy is when we feel sorrow for a person and his or her situation. For example, we might say something like, *"I'm so sorry for your loss."* Sympathy is often communicated in greeting cards or by sending flowers whereby sorrow is expressed. Sympathy tends to be expressed when a situation occurs. Sympathy is also appropriate at *firsts* after a loss, such as a first Mother's Day, Thanksgiving, birthday or anniversary.

Empathy is about asking questions, helping others process their feelings, gaining perspective, acknowledging a situation and communicating understanding. Empathy is acknowledging and discussing a situation without taking on or owning the other person's problem. Examples of questions or statements that are empathetic include:

- *"How does this make you feel?"*
- *"What seems to be the most challenging?"*
- *"Tell me more about ... "*
- *"What's most important to you?"*
- *"How are you going decide about ... ?"*

Empathy and sympathy are two different ways to help comfort and encourage others. I encourage you to place tremendous emphasis on understanding your loved ones and what matters most to them. By understanding their challenges, needs and preferences, you will be better able to meet their care needs and provide the attention and respect your loved ones expect and deserve.

Helping Others Make Life-Altering Decisions

Having already covered extreme situations, I want to discuss common challenges caregivers encounter. Regardless of how obvious or clear-cut something is to you, the reality is that others will see the same situation differently. When discussing issues and encouraging decisions that have the potential to affect a loved one's independence and identity, individuals often come across as being more interested in expressing their opinions and winning others over, rather than trying to reach consensus and find a workable solution to a problem. When stressed, people's behaviors tend to bring out the worst outcome at a time when everyone wants the best solution. To help families communicate effectively and reach an agreement, I suggest a step-by-step process designed to focus more on facts and less on feelings.

1. Accurately Define the Issue — When an issue is vague or too broadly defined, it can be difficult for participants to have a meaningful conversation and reach a resolution. When tackling tough topics, I suggest caregivers start the conversation by defining the issue to be addressed. When defining an issue, avoid opinion statements because they usually suggest that there is only one acceptable outcome. For example, if you say *"Mom and Dad are no longer able to live independently at home,"* the implied solution may be for mom and dad to move. If mom and dad feel strongly about remaining in their home, you are likely to meet tremendous resistance and get nowhere. Instead, define the issue as a question statement. For example, ask *"How are mom and dad's medical conditions making everyday life challenging, and what factors are limiting their ability to live independently in their current home?"* You may also want to explore their preferences and ask them what options to investigate if living alone becomes impractical. Asking questions suggests a willingness to discuss the situation and an openness to explore the areas of concern, consider alternatives, and not be isolated in your viewpoint.

2. Agree Upon the Issue — At the beginning of the conversation, summarize your concern and clarify the issue to be addressed. Ideally, everyone will at least be in agreement on the issue before the discussion begins, so that everyone is working to address the same problem. If

participants go off on tangents, it is easier to redirect people by restating the purpose of this particular discussion. Without agreement, there tends to be confusion and frustration as people find themselves trying to solve different problems. For example, if you embrace the opinion statement above, you would naturally focus your efforts on identifying new living environments you believe to be more suitable for your parents. However, if you focus on the question statement, you would begin by identifying and understanding your parents' limitations and needs.

3. Address the Needs — When an issue is accurately defined as a question statement, the focus becomes answering the question and expressing individual viewpoints. Make sure to spend ample time talking about and prioritizing before jumping to conclusions. By focusing on the needs, whether actual or perceived, conversations tend to be more objective and less subjective. I define needs as the things that are essential to one's health, wellbeing and safety. For example, if a loved one has limited mobility and cannot easily maneuver the steps, there may be a need to have a full bathroom on the first floor. If participants are willing, I suggest coming up with a list of specific needs and prioritizing the items with the care receivers. When families take the time to understand and address their loved ones' needs, a number of suitable options typically emerge.

4. Assess the Options — One of the best ways to find a solution to a problem is to align the care receiver's prioritized needs with the available options — to find the solution that delivers the best match. In the example above, once there is a clear understanding of the needs and what you are trying to accomplish, a logical next step is to consider the various living environments and care options to determine the best option and why. Make sure to look at the pros and cons of each situation and option. If there is a difference of opinion

with the people involved, it can be help to discuss the attitudes, beliefs and values of the care receivers.

5. Agree on a Solution — By addressing steps 1 through 4, multiple solutions often emerge that families find to be suitable. Agree on the solution that appears best or is most acceptable. If the care receivers are of sound mind, the final decision, regardless of whether the caregivers agree or not, is ultimately up to the care receiver. Knowing that, steps 1 through 4 are your chance to try to influence the ultimate solution and share information that may help your loved ones make an informed decision.

Decision Spectrum ᴿᴹ

The Decision Spectrumᴿᴹ is a specific tool I have developed to help families communicate and reach decisions. Let's say you are considering living arrangements for your parent. When you begin to consider and evaluate the various arrangements and the associated lifestyle implications, it helps to think about the situation as a spectrum of options. The spectrum shows a line or continuum with each of the end points representing an extreme position — *Change is Needed* and *No Need for Change.* In the middle, you have a more flexible position or preference — *Change is Imminent or Preferred.* Notice how the words above the line indicate both end points are definitive and absolute.

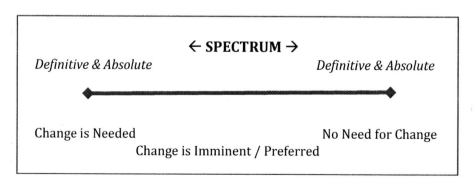

← SPECTRUM →

Definitive & Absolute   *Definitive & Absolute*

Change is Needed   No Need for Change
Change is Imminent / Preferred

How To Use The Decision Spectrum

Step 1: Take out a blank sheet of paper and write the word "Issue:" with a line next to it. On the line, write down the specific issue to be addressed. Remember, write the issue as a question statement, *not* an opinion statement.

ISSUE: _____

Step 2: About two inches below the Issue line draw the Decision Spectrum and label the end points (see the image above). This line represents the spectrum of options that may be available.

Step 3: Ask the participants to indicate where they feel they are along the spectrum, relative to this issue. Make a hash mark along the continuum that represents the opinion of each family member. The hash marks are critical because they can help the participants visualize where everyone is along the spectrum relative to the issue being discussed. This step enables everyone to gain an appreciation for the concerns that will need to be confronted before any type of acceptable agreement can be reached.

Step 4: Ask the question WHY? For example, *"Dad, why do you believe you are fine in the current situation?"* Write down the main points expressed by each person. At the same time, you will have an opportunity to state your concerns. Focus on specific concerns you have, what you believe is important, and why. Make sure to discuss and distinguish between needs and wants.

Step 5: Consider everyone's perspective. Does anything that was said cause anyone to change their position? Remember, this is not about right vs. wrong or winning vs. losing. Keep in mind that a suitable solution accepted by everyone may be somewhere in the middle of the spectrum. Throughout this process, in addition to identifying areas of concern, be sure to acknowledge and celebrate when there is agreement among family members.

Step 6: Now that you have taken the opportunity to consider and understand other family members' perspectives, go back to Step 3 and ask each person if they would change or keep the position of their hash mark. Determine if the gap is narrowed, and if everyone is closer in their thinking.

Step 7: Assuming that the hash marks on the Decision Spectrum are clustered, start working toward specific solutions. Consider the various options that might be available, the pros and cons of each, and work toward a solution that addresses the prioritized needs. Note: It may take more than one discussion to work through the steps and arrive at a solution, and that is okay. Even if you only get to step 2 or 3, it is progress — a step in the right direction.

When applying the Decision Spectrum, do not be surprised if you and your parents are at opposite ends of the spectrum. Regardless of the issue, it can be challenging to realize and understand others' perspectives and needs. It can be frustrating when things seem so obvious to you, but your parents have a different opinion. Remember to take things one day at a time and target small victories while working toward a bigger, more encompassing solution. Also, before you try to influence a decision, think about the repercussions of forcing your opinion on someone else. Consider what is ultimately most important — the relationship or the outcome — and act accordingly.

Needs vs. Wants

People often get so caught up and focused on what they want that they overlook or minimize their needs. How can you tell if something is a need or a want? One simple way is to listen to what someone says. For example, *"I want ... "* People often focus on the things they may have to give up or lose when considering a change. This exercise can often help to surface fears and trepidations. Let's take a moment to clarify the distinction between Needs and Wants.

Needs — Things that are critical to one's health, wellbeing and safety, such as:

- Floor plan/layout is conducive to one's level of mobility
- Necessary care and support services are accessible
- Cost is within one's financial means – ability to pay
- Clean environment
- Safe environment

Wants — Things that are *nice to have.* Often these are things which people have become accustomed to such as:

- Privacy
- Inside parking
- Convenience to beauty parlor
- Convenience to places frequented
- Convenience to family members and friends

A great starting point in determining and differentiating needs and wants is to write them down in a list. Through the process of elimination, prioritize within reason. Your family may find it easier to prepare individual lists and then compare and consolidate the lists into one master list. When it is time to prioritize, I suggest the order of importance be your loved ones' needs first, followed by their wants, then your needs and your wants.

If Only ... After our father passed away and my sister and I decided that a nursing home was best for our mother, we began making the tours and hearing the sales pitches. But we were ill-prepared. We had not discussed priorities, and we found ourselves "in the moment," being influenced by things that were not important. The result? We moved our mother in and out of three different nursing homes for various reasons. The reason we decided on the third (and final) home was because we took the time to write down our needs and wants. By doing this, we were able to understand what was important and quickly move to a suitable solution. We found the perfect spot, and mom lived there for the last two years of her life. We were finally confident that we made the right decision on her behalf and had a clear understanding of what was necessary and acceptable.

Make sure your first list is general enough so you are not trying to force a solution. Even if something sounds obvious, write it down. Start with a general list and narrow down the alternatives. Then determine what really matters before exploring options.

Completing Your List

Needs and Wants lists are great for all lifestyle considerations including dietary, medication and even driving concerns. For example, if you think it is time to intervene or suggest that a parent stop driving, complete the lists. You might find that your parent wants to have the autonomy and independence a car provides; however, when you get down to it, he or she may only drive a few times a week. Thus, the challenge may be to show how alternative methods of transportation can meet his or her need of going to luncheons, the barber or beauty parlor, the doctor, drug store, etc. Also, when giving consideration to needs, give some thought to others who have similar transportation needs. In other words, if your father has a weekly luncheon with someone, maybe that person can pick up your father, thus eliminating the need for him to drive. By identifying the needs and alternatives, people often find that many needs are much easier to address than they might think.

Convincing A Loved One To Accept Help

Your loved one's reluctance to accept help creates conflict and stress for those who are attempting to provide support. However, concerns about a person's health, safety and wellbeing make it appropriate and even necessary to bring up topics that older adults would rather not discuss. A good starting point is to talk about your own feelings, concerns and needs. For example, *"Mom, I am worried about your going up and down the stairs because you might fall and hurt yourself. With your osteoporosis you could get badly hurt. I'd like to talk with you about hiring someone to do the laundry for you, so you do not have to go down to the basement."* At the same time, bring up fears that may not have been expressed, such as, *"This doesn't mean I want you to move to a nursing home. I want to help you stay in your home."* Getting the issues out on the table gives families a chance to discuss them, even though it may be uncomfortable at first. Though it may be simple for you to see a workable solution for someone else, your point of view might not take into consideration the things your loved one is thinking and experiencing.

Occasionally, your loved one may refuse to do something, such as see a doctor. Naturally, you will get frustrated, especially when it's something that seems obvious. When this happens, I recommend:

- Avoid going behind someone's back (e.g., hiring a caregiver, purchasing long-term care insurance.) Instead, have a heart-to-heart talk with your loved one, and encourage them to do something different. In the movie *Driving Miss Daisy*, Dan Ackroyd hired Morgan Freeman behind his mother's back to be her driver. Her response of *"Last I knew I had rights ... "* seemed quite appropriate to me. While he may have had good intentions, I question if he acted appropriately or selfishly.

- Avoid telling your loved one what they need to do. Instead, try making a plea for them to do something for YOU, not for themselves. For example, *"If you refuse to get a personal emergency response system (PERS) for yourself, get it for me so I'm able to sleep instead of being up all night worrying about whether you are okay. If you have a PERS at least I know you can get help at the push of a button. Please mom, do it for me."*

Many times, an aging loved one reacts out of fear. If they appear selfish, they may fear losing your companionship. If you are feeling controlled or influenced by an older adult, it may be time to put your foot down and stop taking orders. Set ground rules and establish boundaries. Know your limits and make sure you do not sacrifice your own life. Also, explore the alternatives.

A Closing Thought

As I alluded to earlier, one of the worst things caregivers can do is try to force someone to do something against their will. Power struggles rarely, if ever, work. Try to be understanding and optimistic at all times. Address a loved one's objections or hesitations creatively, rather than arguing with them.

Throughout this chapter, the focus has been on communication challenges between the care receivers and the caregivers. This is not to suggest that people serving as family caregivers always see eye to eye. Misunderstanding or miscommunication can be devastating to family relationships. Also, sibling rivalry dating back years and years could come up. If you are trying to express yourself and get beyond what has kept you apart, speak frankly — say what you mean, mean what you say, just do not be mean when you say it. Be careful not to come across as though you have all the answers. Remember, people have two ears and only one mouth. Ask questions and be open to another's thoughts and ideas.

If you find yourself in a situation where there is role reversal, realize it can be difficult for loved ones to accept. After all, your parents took care of you, now you are asking them to take on the child role so you can parent them. This can be a tough pill to swallow. Even though roles are reversed because of the caregiving situation, keep in mind your parents are not children, but are in a dependent role due to their care needs. Here are a few words of advice:

1. Be honest and appropriately straight forward.

2. The safety of the care recipient and those around him or her is critical. Realize that your goal of safety may conflict with your parent's goal of independence.

3. If you have siblings, make sure everyone is in agreement on the issues and roles.

4. Talk to your parent in a non-threatening manner.

5. Do not try to force change overnight. Take your time and accept small victories.

6. Do not force your beliefs or wishes on your parent.

KEY LEARNINGS – *Top three findings from this chapter:*

1.

2.

3.

ACTION ITEMS - *Things you want to do or do differently:*

Check when Completed	Action Item	Target Completion Date

*"Only those who avoid love
can avoid grief."*
– John Brantner

8.

Understanding Loss and Grieving

Grief is a normal and expected response to any significant loss, actual or anticipated. In this chapter, I share insight and information to help you make sense of the grieving process and understand what it means to work through loss. While people tend to associate loss and grieving with death, it can encompass much more.

Loss, whether as a result of illness, injury or death, causes a separation between people that matter to one another. For example, if loved ones experience functional loss — physical or cognitive — even though still living, it is quite common for both the caregivers and care receivers to grieve both the loss and the anticipated death. Conditions such as dementia, brain injury and mental illness can be especially challenging because a loved one may be neither clearly present nor clearly absent. Researchers call this "Ambiguous Loss." [117] With cancer, there may be extreme fatigue, which is the loss of strength and stamina, or loss of hair as a result of treatment.

Grieving is an automatic response to loss and is defined as a state of deep mental anguish. Simply stated, it is a process of accepting the unacceptable. It is often expressed through emotions such as sorrow, heartache, pain, distress and misery. The death of a family member leaves a void in life that may never be filled by anyone else. There are no easy answers or quick fixes to help people work through the grieving process. In fact, it is important not to try to rush the normal grief cycle. Down-playing or suppressing your feelings may provide short-term relief; however, there is often long-term unresolved pain.

Life Challenges

For caregivers and care receivers the grieving process often begins when a life-threatening medical condition is diagnosed or incapacity becomes apparent. For many people, grieving is associated with fears. C.S. Lewis once said, *"No one ever told me that grief felt so like fear."* That may include the fear of losing control, being alone, maintaining dignity later in life, ongoing pain and suffering or becoming dependent on others. Additionally, people may fear the inability to cope, leaving loved ones behind, ceasing to exist and even the unknown.

In addition to emotional conflict due to loss, people nearing the end of life often grieve as they anticipate their future death. This is one reason why the spiritual support associated with Hospice care can be so valuable to the dying and their family members. Many people find it helpful to express themselves and discuss aspects of life and death that may be troubling them. For example, some people may have a feeling of being punished or forgotten by God, while others look forward to the end of pain and suffering, and leaving the troubles of this world behind. Regardless of how loved ones grieve, it can be helpful for family and friends to show respect and empathy, and be attentive to their loved ones needs and wishes. One universal, yet often unspoken, wish people have is not to die alone. At the end of life, it is quite important to minimize any pain and suffering, and to maximize comfort and quality of life.

Regardless of the situation, people who are grieving express themselves in many different ways. The range of expression varies from denial or not wishing to discuss the situation, to continuous talking about one's health and future. In terms of physical activity, some people may become overly active and busy as a way to keep their mind off their problems. Others may become inactive finding it hard to get through each new day and being consumed by their problems.

Ways Grief Is Manifested

Some people experience grief in many ways, whereas others only a few. As you and your loved ones grieve, do not be surprised if you notice some of the following signs or indications of grief:

- Absent-minded behavior
- Defensiveness or protectiveness
- Depression
- Inability to concentrate
- Intense feelings of sadness
- Lack of energy and strength

In addition to these more common manifestations of grief, you and your loved ones may experience any or all of the following categories of grief:

- Emotional Grief — Sadness, guilt, loneliness, anger, depression, self-doubt, anxiety, resentment, irritability, etc. Also feelings of hopelessness, helplessness, being overwhelmed, victimized and more.

- Physical Grief — Nausea, tears, sobbing, shock, restlessness, exhaustion, inability to sleep and even wailing. Also, dry mouth, inability to sleep, loss of appetite, and shortness of breath.

- Mental Grief — Confusion, denial, inability to concentrate, need to rationalize and assess one's feelings, sensing that you are in a dream and things are not real, a need for closure, etc.

- Spiritual Grief — Renewed or shaken religious beliefs, feelings of being blessed and at peace, or feelings of being punished. Also, increased confidence or questioning of a higher power, increased prayer and prayer requests, searching for answers and explanation, questioning of what happens to someone's soul after death, etc.

- Social Grief — A need for isolation or withdrawal, dependency on family and friends, rejection or resentment of those offering help and comfort, a need to find distractions, reluctance to ask others for help, a desire to move somewhere else, etc.

Why Grieve?

So why do people grieve? Grieving is a personal expression of how people deal with loss. The following are a few central needs of grief that explain the importance of working through the process:

- " ... to inwardly experience and outwardly express the reality of loss through mourning;

- ... to tolerate the pain of grief while caring for oneself;

- ... to convert the relationship with the lost person from presence to memory, and,

- ... to develop a new self-identity based on life without the person who died, taking on new roles and exploring positive aspects of oneself in the change." [118]

- "... to relate the experience of loss to a context of meaning, telling a story about the loss until it becomes "the story" that makes some sense of it all, teaches some lesson or provides some doorway to continuance; and,

- ... to develop an understanding, enduring support system, which will provide a strengthening brace while healing takes place in the months and years ahead. This support system comprises fellow human beings who will companion the griever and encourage self-compassion whenever a normal resurgence of intense grief occurs." [119]

Rather than coming up with my own eloquent description of grief, I share two of my favorite descriptions of grief. The first is by John Eldredge in his book *Wild at Heart*: [120]

"It was not your fault and it did matter. Oh what a milestone day that was for me when I simply allowed myself to say that the loss of my father mattered. The tears that flowed were the first I'd ever granted my wound, and they were deeply healing. All those years of sucking it up melted away in my grief. It is so important for us to grieve our wound; it is the only honest thing to do. For in the grieving we admit the truth — that we were hurt by someone we loved, that we lost something very dear, and it hurt us very much. Tears are healing. They help to open and cleanse the wound... Grief is a form of validation, it says the wound mattered."

The second description is by C.W. Metcalf and Roma Felible in their book entitled *Lightening Up: Survival Skills for People Under Pressure.* [121]

"We need rest, relaxation, nourishment, and diversions to be replenished from the exhaustion of grief. We need a sense of security, trust, and hope in the future, gained by experiences of being cared for. We need that which will give impetus and direction to life when it seems to

be without meaning. We need lightheartedness, simple pleasures, and humor, which provide balance and relief from stress."

Phases Of The Process

You have probably heard the terms grieving and mourning numerous times, and you may have used them interchangeably, but they are, in fact, different.

- Grieving is an *internal* manifestation individuals go through as they come to accept and work through loss.

- Mourning refers to the *external* demonstration of grieving and includes events and activities that involve a group of people, such as a visitation or funeral.

Grief and mourning are necessary steps in adjusting to the loss of a loved one. The grieving process is about working through loss, coming to accept the loss, and making adjustments in our lives that enable us to move forward. The goal of grieving is not to *get over it,* but to *get through it.* In other words, we do not need to deny the past and pretend the person and our relationship did not matter, in order to renew ourselves and look forward to the future.

There are many different models that explain the stages or phases of the grieving process. A popular five-step model is as follows: Denial, Anger, Bargaining, Depression and Acceptance.[122] The duration of each phase varies from person to person. For some people, each phase may last a few days or weeks each, while for others it may be months. The closer you are to the deceased, the longer or more intense each phase will likely be.

Let's look more closely at a popular grieving model developed by Bowlby and Parkes that reflects four stages.[123]

1. Shock & Disbelief – In this phase, we begin to realize the reality of our loss. Many will have a hard time accepting the facts and will want to hold on to the belief that "it just cannot be." This phase impacts a person's body, mind and soul. Many people will withdraw to protect themselves and re-engage slowly over time.

2. Searching & Yearning – This phase is when people try to understand what has happened and why. People often seek answers. Common thoughts include, *"Why this?" "Why my loved one?" "Why now?" "If only … ,"* and, *"This couldn't have happened."*

3. Disorganization & Despair – During this phase, people may be depressed, appear lazy, absent-minded and indifferent. Commons statements include, *"I just don't care anymore," "I can't go on without him/her,"* and, *"My life is over."*

4. Rebuilding & Healing – At this point, we are becoming accustomed to life without the deceased and are beginning to develop a renewed sense of identity and purpose. During this phase, we work to restructure and reorganize our lives.

Factors That Complicate Grief

Coping with loss can be challenging, as it is not something most people have experience with. Many times in life, people deal with loss through replacement — for example, the family dog dies, and you get a new puppy. As a result, many people have never experienced a significant loss and prolonged grieving.

Loved ones who have played an important role or have significantly influenced your life cannot be replaced and will not be forgotten. People who have minimized grief by pursuing a replacement will find it challenging to know what to do or how to feel when they lose someone who is near and dear. Other factors that can complicate grief include:

- Not being present when a loved one dies.
- A death that occurs suddenly, without anticipation or warning.
- A death that is traumatic or painful.
- A death of a child or younger person.

Whatever your situation, my recommendation is to not rush the grieving process or hold it inside. Get it out. Talk about your feelings with family and friends. Internalizing the pain often makes things worse and prolongs the grieving process. Every situation is unique and everyone handles the grieving process differently. The following are examples of normal responses to grief:

- Keeping busy, managing tasks and details to avoid the reality of a loss.
- Being concerned if you do not break down in tears or feel extreme sadness.
- Being so upset that you are unable to cope for weeks or months.

Abnormal responses include suicidal thoughts and actions that may lead to self-injury. Seek immediate medical attention and the services of a psychologist or psychiatrist in either of these circumstances. Other unhealthy reactions that may indicate a need for professional grief counseling include:

- Postponing grief — indefinitely delaying one's expression of grief.
- Displacing grief — directing intense feelings elsewhere in life.
- Replacing grief — avoiding grief by reinvesting feelings in another relationship.

- Minimizing grief — rationalizing to downplay the impact of loss.
- Somaticizing grief — converting expression of grief into physical symptoms.

Men and women often grieve differently. Women tend to verbalize their emotional responses to grief, and men tend to be more withdrawn and try to exert more control over the areas of their life where control still exists after the loss of a loved one.

Coping Mechanisms

To adjust to loss, people often spend time reminiscing on life and times shared together. We often gain a sense of closure by reflecting on special occasions. Looking through old photos, reading cards and notes, journaling, and spending time in prayer are all examples of coping mechanisms.

Adapting to a loss often requires a focused effort by the survivors to adjust to life without a loved one. As a result of a death, we experience a void in our life that is forever apparent and results in feelings of sadness and loneliness. We are no longer able to visit with a loved one or to talk over the telephone. Special events and holidays are not the same, because a loved one who has played an important role in life is not there to share in the celebration. Flashbacks and vivid memories of loved ones often make a loss more painful and emotional.

In addition to the physical and emotional expressions of grieving, many people express themselves spiritually. Our individual spiritual beliefs are likely to influence how we feel or respond to death. Regardless of our religious background or preference, many of us will turn to prayer and our faith in a higher power as a means of coping and finding strength for the future.

Death may be further complicated as we become more aware of our own mortality and how precious life is. In other words, at a time when we are grieving the loss or death of a loved one, we face our own fears of a terminal illness and the end of life.

When a loved one is no longer physically present, he or she often lives on through a son, daughter and even grandchildren. Mannerisms, expressions, sayings, and behaviors often become apparent in other generations. You may notice a son has eyes just like dad. Or, a daughter has mom's smile.

Other signs or ways of demonstrating grief sometimes include a need to vent feelings, blame others, or get even through legal action or violence. I suggest expressing your emotions and energy in positive ways that can help you move forward. While people cope the best they can, we all need hope for the future. Oftentimes, people simply need to get through today and deal with tomorrow when it gets here, and put the past behind.

While we are all powerless over death, remember that everyone grieves in different ways. Be respectful of how others grieve or otherwise respond to a significant loss. According to researcher J. William Worden, PhD, *"The expected timeframe for full resolution of grief is one to two years, a projected point where natural sadness of having lost will no longer have the initial wrenching quality."* [124]

While few deaths are easy on the survivors, a sudden and painful death can complicate grieving (e.g. suicide, murder or car accident). In these situations, professional counseling can provide needed support to people who struggle to cope with the loss of a loved one.

End-of-Life Considerations

Family members are often shocked when they realize the many tough decisions they face as a result of a terminal illness or death. Two issues many people wish they were better informed about are Hospice Care and Advance Directives. In my book *Engaging While AGING* I address these topics in detail.

Hospice Care — One decision many families face is when to switch from attempts to medically treat or cure an illness, to comfort care and pain management. Many people associate hospice with cancer diagnosis; however, hospice care is designed for people whose life expectancy is limited (projected to be six months or less), and have a medical condition that is beyond trying to find a cure or prolong life. Hospice offers dignified and compassionate comfort care that focuses on life, not illness. Palliative (comfort) care focuses on reducing discomfort or suffering, and improving the quality of life so people can live life to the fullest. As one Hospice Chaplain stated, *"We're not here to hasten death. We're here to make people comfortable. It doesn't mean the individual has given up. It just means that they have resolved themselves to the fact that they know this disease is going to end up taking their life. They just want to have time to really live before they die."* [125]

Advance Directives are legal documents that let health care professionals and others know one's wishes for medical treatment, in the event the person becomes unable to speak for him or herself. Advance Directive documents are available free of charge through your state. For information on state specific advance directive documents visit: www.partnership forcaring.org — a service of the National Hospice and Palliative Care Organization. If your loved one's advance directives appoint you to make decisions on their behalf should they be unable, you must know their wishes in order to honor their wishes. For each of the different advance directives, I share a few questions which you need to be able to answer:

- A Living Will (Living Will Declaration) expresses a person's wishes about his or her health care. Each state has an approved or standard version of a Living Will form. The National Hospice and Palliative Care Organization website has a link to each state form and instructions. To download the a form visit www.caringinfo.org/stateaddownload.

  The Living Will form is used to express a person's wishes about life-sustaining medical treatment should he or she become terminally ill, unable to communicate or declared permanently unconscious. It does not require anyone to act on their behalf. By indicating choices regarding life support, family members and your medical doctor avoid much of the guess work.

  A copy of a Living Will is typically requested when an organization such as a hospital or long-term care center begins providing health care services. The document serves as instruction to health care personnel regarding his or her desired treatment. A Living Will can be a valuable tool as it eliminates the need for family members to struggle with difficult medical decisions and determine what heroics, if any, are appropriate.

- Health Care Power of Attorney — This form, also known as a Durable Power of Attorney for Health Care, is used to appoint someone as an agent to make health care decisions on a loved one's behalf. The appointed person makes decisions if the loved one is unable to do so because of a terminal illness or temporary or permanent unconsciousness. Check a state's requirement to make sure the DPOA is properly executed. For example, to be considered valid in the State of Ohio, the completed form must be signed by two witnesses or be notarized. If you are appointed by a loved one to make health care decisions on his or her behalf, make sure you discuss and understand the person's wishes, such as:

o Does your loved one want to be resuscitated should his or her heart stop?

o Does your loved one want to be hooked up to a respirator, feeding tube or other life-support device if it is necessary to sustain life?

o How does your loved one feel about withdrawing life-sustaining treatment that could prolong the dying process?

o What are your loved one's feelings about medical treatments and surgeries that could prolong life?

Besides addressing life-sustaining treatment that may prolong the dying process, other issues, such as cardiac resuscitation (CPR) and organ donation may be addressed. Resuscitation orders and organ donation may also be addressed in stand-alone documents or be indicated on a person's driver's license.

- Do Not Resuscitate (DNR) — A DNR order tells health care professionals not to attempt to revive someone who stops breathing or whose heart stops. This means that doctors, nurses and emergency medical personnel will be instructed not to attempt emergency resuscitation or CPR. While DNR is the commonly used term, the term can be misleading as it suggests an attempt at resuscitation will be successful. Many people believe the term DNAR standing for *"Do Not Attempt Resuscitation"* is more appropriate. Either way, DNR essentially means to allow a natural death. The term that I prefer is AND standing for *"Allow Natural Death."* Realizing the thought of withholding treatment can be quite difficult for challenging for caregivers, you might find comfort in thinking of it as allowing a natural death to occur.

- Organ and Tissue Donation is yet another choice for people to make and is a way to save the lives of others. Approximately 100,000 people are on national waiting lists to receive one or more needed organs. People who choose to become an organ donor may be able to give life to someone else by donating their kidneys, liver, heart, lungs and other body parts. Thousands of people also need tissue donations such as eyes, skin and bone. Family members may find comfort in dealing with the pain of loss knowing a loved one may be able to help save someone else. If you or your loved ones wish to become an organ or tissue donor, contact your state Bureau of Motor Vehicles and sign your state's form to become an organ donor. Your driver's license will indicate your choice to become a donor. You can also make your wishes known in your Advance Directives or by signing up with the Organ and Tissue Donor Registry in your state.

Guardianship

There is one additional legal issue I believe merits mention. If a person with a serious medical condition or traumatic injury is deemed incompetent by expert evaluation, guardianship may be appropriate if there is No Power of Attorney. If your loved one has not made arrangements granting someone else the authority to manage his or her affairs and make decisions on his or her behalf, you might speak with an attorney to determine if pursuing guardianship may be wise.

A Closing Thought

For caregivers, it is natural to grieve the loss of loved ones before, during and after the actual time of death. While grieving is often most apparent during the active dying phase and upon death, do not be surprised if you find yourself grieving the losses associated with disease and disability.

When a loved one dies, grieving is most apparent over the first six to 12 months. Also, any *firsts* such as a first Mother's Day, first Thanksgiving, birthday or anniversary without your loved one can be especially difficult.

Once you have experienced a death, do not be alarmed by comments that seem insensitive. It will happen. Remember how awkward you were when one of your friends was dealing with a loss and you were not sure what to do or say. I know that when both of my parents died, I felt helpless. I did not know what I should do. My life was turned upside down, yet, the world continued to revolve in spite of my loss.

The emotional wounds left by death take time to heal. It is becoming more and more common for people who are grieving to talk with a professional counselor or participate in an aftercare support group to help deal with loss and grief. You might contact your religious leader, local funeral home director or a local hospice to learn about options available in your community.

A word of caution — if you are married or have children, do not shut them out and carry the entire burden on your shoulders. Children are often more perceptive than we care to admit. They also have a need to understand. There are some great children's books available at bookstores and libraries to help children understand death and dying.

KEY LEARNINGS – *Top three findings from this chapter:*
1.
2.
3.

ACTION ITEMS - *Things you want to do or do differently:*		
Check when Completed	*Action Item*	*Target Completion Date*

"When someone you love becomes a memory,
the memory becomes a treasure."
– Author Unknown

9.

Preparing for End-of-Life

Accepting the fact that a loved one is dying or has died is always difficult. Combine that with feelings of guilt, sadness, loneliness, agitation and more -- and chances are, you will find yourself on an emotional roller coaster. For most people, dying is a process. Deterioration can be slow or rapid. When death becomes a likely reality, family members often reprioritize the things they do and how they spend their time. The movie *Dad,* which I referenced in Chapter 2, offers a wonderful and powerful portrayal of the life and death experience, and it shares perspectives I believe caregivers may find helpful to understand early in their journey.

Death Is A Reality Of Life

Death is one of the most difficult realities we all face in life. People are said to handle death in ways similar to how they approach life. Some people want to isolate and approach death in a private manner while others want to be surrounded by loved ones. Some may be more reserved, others more expressive. There is no right or wrong way. While this may seem over-simplified, I believe family members can process the death of a loved one in one of two ways:

1. Grieve the death
2. Celebrate the life

It is my hope that your loved ones have lived long and fulfilling lives, and that in the midst of your grieving you will be able to celebrate their lives. While old age does not make death any easier, it is something people expect as loved ones reach their 70's and 80's. In the case of a premature or unexpected death, do not be surprised if you may find the grieving to be more intense. Unexpected deaths can be extremely heart-wrenching because family has not had a chance to prepare or say goodbye. When grieving an abrupt death, it can take time to work through your feelings — whether they are of confusion, guilt or anger. Regardless of the situation, it takes time to heal wounds.

If your parent passes away after battling an illness or disease, it can be comforting to know he or she has finally been relieved from pain and suffering. As part of the healing process, spend time reflecting on your parent's life, reliving wonderful memories and appreciating the traditions in your family. During these emotional flashbacks, my hope is that more of your tears are of joy instead of sadness.

As I look back, one my biggest regrets has to do with my dad's death. If only someone had given me some insight, and I had known better. My dad had been fighting lymphoma leukemia for a couple years, and on his 79th birthday, he became rather delirious after catching what I thought was a common cold. The cold turned out to be pneumonia. Over the next two weeks, he became quite agitated and began doing and saying things I had never observed before. While I visited him each day, it was very difficult seeing him restrained for his own safety and being with him when his behavior was so unlike the man I knew and loved. It got to the point where I just could not face him in that condition. Frankly, it was scary and sad. While I never gave up hope that he would pull through, days later, the doctor called to tell us he would not make it through the night. I chose not to be by his side because I was afraid of death, did not know what to expect and just could not cope. From all that I had seen on television and in movies I viewed death as being a painful and horrific experience. That night in March 1997 he passed away. As I look back, I wish I would have been by his side... holding his hand and telling him how much I loved him.

As for our mom, she had been challenged by dementia for years. She lived at the Alois Alzheimer's Center (www.Alois.com) in a marvelous place where everyone there loved her. On Thanksgiving weekend of 2001, I got the call. She was deteriorating rapidly. When I arrived it was apparent that many of her bodily functions were shutting down. She was on oxygen and was taking huge, gaspy breaths. I sat down at mom's bedside and even though she was unconscious, I thanked her for a wonderful life and reflected on a few fond memories, told her that I loved her and I always would. After that I told her that it was okay, almost as if I gave her permission to die. Finally, I told her she was going to a most wonderful place. She immediately began to breathe easier and within minutes, she died at the age of 70. Words cannot describe what a beautiful experience it was to see her released from her suffering. I only wish I had been by my dad's bedside when he died.

I share my story for a couple of reasons:

1. To help you gain perspective to determine what is right for you. If, given the chance to be by your loved one's side, think through what might be right for you.

2. To offer a perspective on death and dying. Prior to my parents' death, I had no any idea what to expect.

Death Considerations

Many people struggle to focus their attention on the many issues that arise immediately following a loved one's death. When a death occurs, whether sudden or expected, family members can quickly find themselves emotionally and physically exhausted. To help reduce some of the stress that tends to occur upon death, many families choose to pre-plan funeral arrangements. The stories I have heard from people who have pre-planned funerals with loved ones are always positive. What initially seems to focus on the specific plans often goes off on tangents where reminiscing brings welcomed joy.

Whether loved ones pre-plan their arrangements or surviving family members make the decisions upon death, decisions tend to be based on a person's religious preferences, cultural traditions and personal wishes. Your funeral director and religious leader can help you work through the process and coordinate the arrangements. While there is a lot to consider when a loved one dies, at a minimum, it may be helpful to give advance consideration to the following three issues:

1. The Remains – The typical choices are earth burial of the body in a casket, earth burial of an urn or box containing a loved ones ashes (cremains), scattering of a loved one's ashes, or entombment. Assuming your loved ones are living and of sound mind, my recommendation is to ask them. If a loved one has passed, and you are uncertain of his or her wishes, they may be stated in his or her Will. When this conversation recently came up with my wife after having attended a friend's funeral, I was surprised to learn her

preference for burial, just as she was surprised to hear my preference for cremation.

2. Obituary (also known as a death notice): Obituaries appear in the local newspaper and share information about the deceased and the funeral arrangements. A basic obituary includes the name of the deceased, surviving family members, a brief summary of work, military service or community involvement, date and time of the service and other arrangements. Many obituaries also designate an organization or charity to receive financial gifts in memory of the deceased. A standard death notice is basically a classified advertisement and is billed at a per-line charge by most newspapers. You may wish to write a more detailed life review that can be shared in a bulletin and handed out at the service.

3. Service Arrangements: It can be helpful to request copies of programs from recent funeral services to give you an idea of what other people have done. You will want to consider if you would like anyone to share a scripture reading or story. Are there certain songs or music you would like played or performed? For the person presiding over the ceremony, are there certain things you would like to encourage him or her to say? Will someone from the family or a close friend speak on behalf of the family? Do not hesitate to ask representatives at a funeral home any and all questions you have.

What To Do And Who To Call

When a person dies, there are a number of issues that need to be addressed, some requiring immediate attention. The following provides insight to the purpose and implications behind many of those tasks. Depending on your religious beliefs, there may be additional considerations not mentioned here. If loved ones have pre-arranged their funerals, many of these steps may already be addressed.

Death at a Private Residence — If a loved one is found dead at a private residence, 911 should be called. Emergency medical services (EMS) and the police will respond to the residence as each has a separate and distinct role.

- Role of EMS — EMS personnel can make a determination about death; however, only a medical doctor can pronounce a person dead and sign a death certificate. If a person is critically ill or is having a medical episode, EMS personnel are required to try to save the person's life unless a Do Not Resuscitate order is immediately available or is on file. If your loved one has a DNR, you can contact the local police department to inquire how to have it noted in the 911 system.

- Role of the Police — The police secure the person's residence and contact both the coroner's office and the next of kin. Initially, the residence must be treated like a crime scene until it is determined otherwise. If there is any possible suspicion about the cause of death, such as bruises, cuts or burns, appropriate action will be taken. The police will also complete a deceased person's report, and a supervisor will likely respond as well.

  o The police will call the coroner's office and provide information such as the age of the deceased, any known medical history, medications and information believed to be pertinent to the death. Based on the information provided, the coroner's office will decide if they need more information and/or if a medical exam is deemed to be necessary. The coroner's office ultimately decides if there is any suspicion surrounding the death and if they need to take the body.

- o The police will also make every effort to contact next of kin. They will typically look for an address book near the telephone, contact information on the refrigerator, or see if ICE numbers are programmed into the deceased's cell phone (ICE stands for In Case of Emergency). They may also contact neighbors for family contact information. The police will stay at the scene with the body until either the coroner takes the body or the family is contacted and arrangements can be made with a local funeral home to take the body.

- Death at a Nursing Home or Hospital — If a loved one dies at a nursing home, assisted living facility or hospital, medical staff will respond by contacting the family and reporting the death with the local authorities.

Regardless of where a death occurs, a medical doctor is required to pronounce a person dead. Assuming the deceased is not already at a medical center where a medical doctor is available, the funeral home that takes the body will go to a local hospital emergency department where the doctor will likely come out to the vehicle and make the formal pronunciation.

If your loved one has not made pre-arrangements, consider which funeral home you would like to handle the arrangements. Consider the following when making a selection:

- Responsiveness and timely follow-up to your telephone calls. Someone is typically on call 24 hours a day and should be able to return your call promptly.

- Positive reputation from family members, friends, neighbors, caregivers, place of worship, etc.

- Licensure and professional designation or affiliation (e.g. National Funeral Directors Association).

Additional Considerations:

1. Notify Friends and Relatives: People usually find that contacting friends and relatives can be an extremely emotional task. Don't hesitate to ask a family friend to make some calls on your behalf.

2. Notify Your Loved One's Attorney: This is important for a number of reasons. First, if there is any question about arrangements or authority to make decisions, the deceased's attorney should have the necessary legal documents (e.g., Will, Power of Attorney) to answer those questions. The attorney can advise of any special wishes, concerns or suggestions. The attorney may also offer to notify your loved one's bank, at which point accounts and access to a safety deposit box may be restricted.

3. Meet with Funeral Home: Usually within 24 hours of a death, you should meet with the funeral home representative to begin making arrangements. Funeral directors are valuable resources who serve as advisors and coordinators of the logistical issues, so do not hesitate to ask any and all questions you have. During your meeting or initial phone conversation, you will be expected to provide information, including the deceased's full name, address, social security number, place of birth, place of death, military service, and more, so they can file the appropriate paper work with the local government agencies. Also, they are likely to require signatures on a number of documents and describe the process over the next few days.

If you have not pre-planned the funeral, be prepared to discuss the following:

- What is the preferred handling of the body (*e.g. earth burial, cremation*)

- Would you like to a have a visitation the evening before the actual ceremony?
- Is there a particular place you would like to hold the funeral or memorial service (e.g. church, synagogue, mosque)?
- Who would you like to perform the ceremony (e.g. religious leader, funeral director)?
- What is the availability of the facility and the person to perform the ceremony?
- Would you like the body prepared for viewing?
- If an earth burial is planned, does the family already have cemetery plots?
- Will there be a graveside service and burial?
- Would you like the funeral home to handle the gravestone arrangements?
- Will the family be receiving guests either before or after the service?
- Would you like to a have private service inviting only family and select friends?
- Who from your family will contribute to or write the obituary? How much help do you want/need from the funeral director for this?
- Is there a charity you would like to designate for memorial contributions to be made in remembrance of the deceased?
- Would you like the funeral home to take care of floral arrangements? If so, do you have any flower preferences?
- Would you like the funeral home to take care of honorariums of the person conducting the memorial service, any musicians or organists, vocalists, etc?
- How many death certificates will you need?

4. Meet with Person Performing the Ceremony — The person performing the ceremony can help you with your selections, including:

- What readings you would like
- What musical selections you would like, and how they will be performed (e.g., vocalist, organ, piano, CD)
- Would you like someone to speak on behalf of the family, and if so, whom?
- Are there specific things you would like to be included in the remarks?
- Are you planning a graveside service following a funeral?
- Will there be pall bearers? Who?

If uncertain when planning a service, a great starting point is to request copies of bulletins of other memorial services. If not available, draft a simple outline. If appropriate, consider coordinating and/or hosting a luncheon or dinner for family, out-of-town guests and close friends.

Years ago, I was driving down the road, and I saw a bumper sticker that caught my eye. It read "Let's put the FUN back in FUNeral". I couldn't agree more. In fact, my mother passed away a couple months after I saw the bumper sticker and that is the approach we took. Sure, we went through a grieving process that included crying, being extremely sad, etc. But, to make it a "celebration" of her life, we conjured up and shared the happy and fun memories at her funeral... we even poked a little fun at mom. We knew she was laughing up there with us ... not slapping our hands. Please note: there is a big difference between being disrespectful and having fun. We knew we had successfully celebrated her life in a tactful, upbeat way when those in attendance laughed more than cried.

Whichever road you choose is fine. However, just realize that funerals do not have to be entirely somber.

Death Certificate

As you may have guessed, a death certificate is similar to a birth certificate. Just as a birth certificate was necessary to obtain a Social Security number, validate identity when enrolling in school, etc., a death certificate is necessary for the following reasons:

- To apply for Social Security Benefits for the surviving spouse
- To apply for retirement funds, deferred salary, accrued vacation pay, unpaid bonuses, commissions, stock options, etc.
- To initiate a claim and collect on insurance benefits
- To transfer investments (Stocks, Bonds, IRA's, etc.) for estate matters

Four to five death certificates will usually suffice; however, if a person has not consolidated their financial assets, such as stocks and bonds, into a managed account, it may be necessary to have individual copies for each institution or company for which assets are held.

According to a 2004 New York Times article entitled *Death and the City*, reporter Wilson H. Beebe Jr. explains dying in New York City can be challenging. Beebe writes, *"... something must be done with you when you die in New York, and that something requires a document. At some point, your name and Social Security number must cross a Health Department desk. Without a certified death certificate, survivors cannot begin probate on a will, make claims on life insurance policies, apply for Social Security benefits, or perform a host of other tasks involving the business of life."* [126] He continues to state that because of New

York's antiquated death registration system, it can take two to six months to get a death certificate. Also, there is only one vital records office in the city. Although the city plans to develop an electronic system to expedite the process, no deadlines have been set. I share this story as you may want to ask the funeral director handling arrangements for your loved one about any special considerations you might want to be aware of in your city or state.

How To Help

After a death occurs, family members may need some assistance, whether they immediately recognize it or not. The following is a list of some things others can help you with. Likewise, when friends experience a death in the family, these are things you can do for them.

- Grocery shopping: Invariably, you will need food, beverages and other supplies. Consider everything from toilet paper and paper products for the kitchen, to snack foods, sandwich items, soft drinks and coffee.

- Make phone calls: Many people will need to be informed that a loved one has died. Consider asking a close family member or friend to contact certain people on your behalf to notify them of the death and funeral arrangements.

- Prepare for guests: If you expect out-of-town guests, consider transportation and lodging arrangements. Also, consider asking a friend to help clean your house so it is presentable for company.

Do not hesitate to ask for support after the initial week or two of support. Families tend to receive a tremendous amount of support (e.g. visits, cards, flowers) over the 7-10 days after death. As a result, the two to four weeks after a death is a time when people often struggle the most. It is as this point when friends, neighbors and co-workers are back to life as before.

Families find themselves dealing with a number of administrative (e.g. legal and financial) issues at this time. Many people comment that they are still acutely aware of their recent loss, and at the same time are amazed that the world continues to revolve and people are going about day-to-day life. This may be a time to reach out for support and encouragement from friends.

Also, when the funeral or memorial service is over and you think you can finally relax, you realize that there is a lot more to do. There are estate matters that need to be addressed, arrangements that need to be made for a gravestone, thank you notes to be sent to people for their flowers and gifts, and do not forget about the tax return that will need to be filed for any income earning or received during your parent's final year.

An often overlooked, yet challenging, aspect of death is handling the distribution of a loved one's personal items. It can be quite difficult to go through a loved one's belongings and make decisions about what to keep, sell, donate and dispose. Most of us have accumulated a lot of stuff over the years. Practically speaking, the deceased often leave a lot of work for the surviving family members. Spiritually speaking, you cannot take it with you and people will not remember you for your possessions. According to friends who have handled thousands of estates over the years, there are stages that family members go through. Initially, families only keep special items that were near and dear to their loved one (e.g. a special antique, piece of art work, a vase, photos, etc.) Then after about three years, people are able to dispose of things that have been stored away in their basement unused for a period of time.

When a loved one dies, it can be extremely difficult to feel optimistic about the future, but know you can ask your friends, family and professionals for support.

A Closing Thought

Death should not be a lonely, painful or traumatic experience for people and their families. Always strive to ensure your loved ones are comfortable and able to maintain their dignity. Everyone responds to death differently. For an older person, factors that often play a significant role include their previous exposure to death, their faith and their personality. Common reactions often include:

- Acceptance or denial
- Peace or anger
- Calm, fear or even guilt

Know that everyone grieves differently. Many people need time and space before they are able to go back to everyday life. Remember, there is no right or wrong way. Do not be afraid to seek professional counseling. When my mother died, I realized I was alone, and for the first time in my life, totally responsible for everything I did. Because of her dementia, my mother did not recognize me during her last years, but it was different once she passed away – I was depressed. I realized I had issues and concerns I had never acknowledged but that needed to be addressed. Also, in addition to taking care of yourself, do not neglect your family. Often people fail to recognize other family members are also impacted directly and indirectly from a death.

KEY LEARNINGS – *Top three findings from this chapter:*

1.

2.

3.

ACTION ITEMS - *Things you want to do or do differently:*

Check when Completed	Action Item	Target Completion Date

*"I would want my legacy to be that
I was a great son, father and friend."*
Dante Hall

10.

Ensuring Lasting Memories

Think about your parent's life, and you can quickly find yourself immersed in a sentimental journey. With the hustle and bustle of life, many people do not spend adequate time capturing memories. Then something happens and it is too late. I have a simple recommendation. Starting now, think about how you can make the most of each and every day.

I have heard it a thousand times — someone is hospitalized or diagnosed with an illness, and suddenly the entire family is reevaluating and reprioritizing everything in life. People start making time for things that were previously overlooked. When a crisis occurs, the reality of life and death often sets in and people realize what is most important in life.

How can you make the most of each new day? Do you find your conversations center around news, weather and sports, as opposed to life? Are there certain memories you would like to preserve forever? I suggest reading the book *Tuesdays with Morrie* by Mitch Albom. I found this book about life's simple lessons to be life-changing. The book is about a professor who has ALS (Lou Gehrig's disease). During the last year of the professor's life, he and a former student get together every

Tuesday to talk about life. The topic of discussion for each get together is determined in advance, and the conversations and lessons are always fascinating. So much wisdom, it's incredible.

It is sad that many people simply never take the time to tap into the wisdom and life experiences of loved ones. Spending time with your loved one reminiscing about the past can be a most rewarding experience.

- Imagine what life must have been like before television, VCRs/DVDs, Velcro, microwave ovens, computers and fast food? How the world has changed over the past century!

- Imagine what it would have been like having your milk and eggs delivered fresh to your doorstep.

- Imagine what it must have been like living through WWI, WWII or the Great Depression?

Especially after the September 11th tragedy, people realize life cannot be taken for granted. Tomorrow is not guaranteed. With that in mind, are there things you want to say? Questions you want to ask? Things you would like to do?

Simple Things To Do

Death is uncertain because people never know when, how, or where it will strike. To families with aging parents, I suggest a few things. At your next family gathering, whether it is a birthday, holiday or other occasion, consider the following:

- Pull Out a Camera and Take Extra Photos. Once our father passed away, my sister realized that she never had a picture of Gramps and her youngest daughter, even though she had a picture of Gramps alone with her other two children. Unfortunately, it was too late. Photographs and videos are memories you can cherish forever. Therefore, do not wait until a loved one has passed before you realize you have not captured certain memories on film. Take a minute now to think which pictures you might cherish that you do not already have.

At your next gathering, pull out a video camera and turn it on. You do not need to tell your mom and dad that you are capturing memories to enjoy once they have passed away. Rather, use it as an opportunity to ask your parent's questions about their life, childhood, how they met, and more. Ask about how you were as a child, what they remember most, your first words, and other fond memories. You will be glad you did. It is always nice to be able to hear someone's voice long after they are gone.

The following is one of my favorite Dear Abby columns:

"Dear Abby: During my mother's fight with breast cancer, she was in and out of hospitals. My sister made a 3-by-4 foot collage of old photographs of family, friends and places that Mom loved to visit. This collage went with her from hospital room to hospital room for the duration of her illness.

It served to remind everyone that Mom was once a vibrant lady with a rich, full life, who was loved by all the people pictured. She was cheered up by it and it served to "humanize" her to the myriad of doctors, nurses, aides and technicians who treated her.

Now that Mom is gone, the collage is hung in a prominent place in our family home. It serves as a constant reminder of how much we love and miss her.

- Dave in Ohio.

Dear Dave: I'm sure your sister's masterpiece is a treasure, and will continue to be considered so by future generations." [127]

For your loved one's next birthday or anniversary, create a video of their life including sequential pictures from childhood to the present. Ask a local camera shop about transferring pictures to a video. You can also add their favorite music. Not only is this a great present for your loved one now, but it is also a present you will treasure for life once they have passed.

- Talk from your Heart. As family, there is a natural tendency to assume that you are loved by one another though the words may rarely be spoken. All too often in this fast-paced world, people take so much for granted. Make sure to tell your loved ones how much you appreciate them and all they have done for you.

Take the time to say what is in your heart before it is too late. The words *I love you* are powerful and need to be said and heard by everyone. Though many people use these words as a salutation, it is more heartfelt to look a parent or loved one in the eyes and tell them *"I love you."* For people who do not express their feelings much, especially men, it can be difficult to say *I love you*, but I recommend working toward it.

You can also honor your parents by scheduling a dinner, inviting family and close friends and asking each person to say a few words. Hold a family *Roast* on a birthday or anniversary, and share fond memories and humorous occasions. Or, as my wife's family does on Christmas, make your gift to each other a letter about fond memories. Most people already have enough stuff, so instead of a present, write a letter of recollection and appreciation or make a list of your top 10 memories.

In the book *Tuesdays with Morrie*, Morrie talks about how unfortunate it is that once someone dies, friends start sharing wonderful stories and memories about the person.

Morrie questioned why we have to wait to say nice things about a person until they have died. He also indicated how unfortunate it is that the person about whom the nice things are being said, isn't there to hear them.

- Ask Questions. I always hear people say that they have heard a particular story a hundred times; however, when it comes time to repeat it, they are at a loss for words. If there are stories of significant interest, write them down or videotape your parent delivering her favorite story, so you capture her expressions and mannerisms. Also, as in the case of my parents, do you look at their wedding album without a clue of who anyone is? Rather than trying to recall if someone might be a family member, friend, neighbor or business associate, go through photo albums with your parent and write down peoples' names, relationship and places.

If your parent has antiques, collectibles or other items of sentimental value, make sure to ask about the history, significance and value. Someone once told me that there is a story behind every antique. Do you know the stories associated with your loved one's antiques and collectibles? Remember to write down what your parents or loved ones tell you.

Take the time to document a loved one's life. You will be amazed at how much you did not know and how much you learn. The following is a list of simple questions to get you started:

- What is something you always wanted to do, but never have? Why?
- What is something specific you vividly remember doing as a child?
- Where did you grow up? How did your parent end up there?

- Where did you go to school? What are some fond memories? Do you still keep in touch with any former classmates?

- Who were your best friends at different stages of your life? Do you have their contact information?

- Where have you lived?

- How did you meet mom/dad? Was it love at first site?

- What do you remember most about dating? How long did you date? What kind of things did you do on dates?

- How and when did your dad propose to your mom? Did she say yes right away?

- What is one thing you regret never doing?

- What is most valuable lesson learned in life and how did you learn it?

- What do you consider to be your biggest achievement? Why?

- What is your fondest memory? Why?

- How would you like to be remembered?

- What do you want your great-grandchildren to know about you?

If you are like most people, you will be astonished as to how little you know or are able to recall about your loved ones. If possible, create a resume or other list of work history, military service, honors and recognition, involvement in clubs, organizations, and other affiliations.

This information can also be great to reference when writing an obituary or preparing remarks to celebrate your loved one's life at their funeral.

- Places of residence
- Places of education
- Military service and honors

- Favorite hobbies
- Club memberships
- Favorite songs
- Favorite artists
- Favorite vacation spots
- Special honors or awards

Just as many people take photographs on vacations and other events, take your own trip down memory lane with your loved one. Reminiscing about the past and of fond memories can be great therapy! Think about it. Who do you know that does not like talking about themselves and sharing insight into life?

As my dad's health was declining, it struck me that my parent's had not been away on vacation for a couple of years. I asked dad about going somewhere and he indicated he would not be able to cope. I then asked if they would consider going away if my wife and I went with them. I vividly remember my parent's excitement. They chose to go to the Greenbrier, a resort they first visited on their honeymoon in 1959. It was an amazing experience. They shared so many fun stories. It was great being with them at a place that was quite significant to both of them. Consider if there is a place you might visit that with your loved ones that might be especially meaningful.

- Create a Family Tree. Trust me, it is a lot easier to do with the input of someone that knows first-hand. Even when someone is knowledgeable, it can be difficult to go back more than a generation or two. If your family has a cemetery plot, you might want to contact the main office at the cemetery to obtain information about each relative that is buried there. Information often includes birth and death dates, cause of death, full name, occupation and more.

My father always seemed a bit sad on his birthday and I always thought he was having a tough time getting older. Upon his death, we obtained records from the office staff at the cemetery where other family members had been buried. I learned that my grandfather died two days before my dad's 9th birthday, and was buried on my dad's birthday. While some might be astonished by this story, remember that many older people are very private about their lives, even to their own family. While I knew his dad passed away when he was nine, I did not know the proximity to my dad's birthday or that my grandfather was only in his forties when he passed.

You might find it helpful to visit a website such as www.Ancestry.com or www.FamilySearch.org for more information about family history. Likewise, you might search the web for a program that will enable you to put together an actual family tree. Using a program can be helpful, especially if you come from a large family or if step relations are involved.

In addition to the ideas suggested, you might consider hiring a personal historian to help you compile materials and recordings to create a legacy project. With many boomers exploring and document their family histories to leave a legacy for future generations, a new career field has emerged. Personal historians can help you research and organize materials, and facilitate recording sessions to capture loved one's sharing stories. In addition to creating multimedia stories, they can also help with writing memoirs. From low tech to high tech, lasting memories are sure to become family heirlooms.

Estate Matters

There is often legacy in personal belongings, especially items of sentimental value (e.g., engagement ring, antiques, artwork, photo albums, collectables). To help avoid family feuds, I suggest you encourage your loved ones to indicate their intentions clearly. If a loved one mentions they want you to have something, ask them to state it in their Will or write you a letter. Bottom line, if there are items over which siblings are likely to fight or feel resentment, encourage your parents to spell it out in order to avoid conflict. When siblings or relatives live in different parts of the country, this can also help avoid the *first-come-first-served* mentality. If a person arrives at a parent's house and starts taking things he or she wants before other family members have a chance to express an interest, it may be too late. Believe it or not this happens.

I was fortunate to receive a few special items from my father, including a watch he received when he graduated from law school, and a painting he received from a dear friend. Unfortunately, once he passed away, and I attempted to share the significance, I found myself unable to recall the specifics around both items. I am now frustrated to realize that I will be unable to share the heritage with my children. It would have been so easy to write down what he told me.

A Closing Thought

All too often family members are so physically close to a loved one that they take for granted that they know the intimate details of a loved one's life. Then, when the time comes to write the obituary, you may discover you cannot recall the details like you thought you would. While it is natural to think you know a tremendous amount about a parent's life, people often do not realize they were not yet alive during their parents' first 20 or 30 years. Until your teenage years, you were too young to recall any details or specifics. It always seems the most recent experiences are the memories that are so vivid, yet they represent such a small part of a loved one's life.

Do not take life for granted. Take time to capture special memories and make every interaction count! Be prepared for some good laughs, and tears of joy and sorrow.

I sincerely hope that the material presented throughout this book helps to prepare you for the journey ahead. When it comes to caregiving, people who have never been a caregiver quickly realize they know very little about what to expect, what to do, and more. When I tell my children to go out and do their best, I am reminded they have typically had some sort of training, coaching and time to develop their skills. Therefore, contrary to popular opinion, caregivers do the best they don't know how to do. I wish you the best as you apply the information, insight, and inspiration from this book and make a difference in the lives of those you have the privilege to serve.

Too many people serving as family caregivers are struggling unnecessarily. Assuming you have found this book to be a blessing, I ask that you would please recommend *CAREGIVING Ready or Not* to your family, friends, neighbors and coworkers. As I mentioned in Chapter 1, everyone will be impacted by caregiving at some point in their life. If I can be of assistance, my contact information is available at www.Caregiving.CC. I pray that your journey will be rewarding.

Let me close by sharing excerpts from an e-mail I received in 2002 that I believe were originally written by Andy Rooney.

I'VE LEARNED....

- That being kind is more important than being right.

- That I can always pray for someone when I do not have the strength to help him in some other way.

- That sometimes all a person needs is a hand to hold and a heart to understand.

- That under everyone's hard shell is someone who wants to be appreciated and loved.

- That the Lord didn't do it all in one day. What makes me think I can?

- That to ignore the facts does not change the facts.

- That I cannot choose how I feel, but I can choose what I do about it.

KEY LEARNINGS – *Top three findings from this chapter:*
1.
2.
3.

ACTION ITEMS - *Things you want to do or do differently:*

Check when Completed	*Action Item*	*Target Completion Date*

References

1. The Rosalynn Carter Institute - http://rci.gsw.edu.
2. *Caregivers | Undervalued Resources* - Editorial. The Cincinnati Enquirer, Oct. 28, 2002.
3. M. Hobson. *Paying for Parents and Kids*. ABC News. Retrieved April 18, 2006 from http://abcnews.go.com/GMA/print?id=1813409.
4. *Health Aging Improving and Extending Quality of Life Among Older Adults, At A Glance: 2009*. The Centers for Disease Control and Prevention. Retrieved March 13, 2009 from www.cdc.gov/nccdphp/publications/aag/pdf/healthy_aging.pdf.
5. *Caregiving in the U.S. 2004*. National Alliance for Caregiving and AARP. Retrieved September 3, 2005 from www.caregiving.org/data/04finalreport.pdf.
6. *Families Care: Alzheimer's Caregiving in the United States. 2004*. Alzheimer's Association and National Alliance for Caregiving. Retrieved September 3, 2005 from www.alz.org/national/documents/report_familiescare.pdf.
7. See reference 5
8. Ibid
9. J.T. Bond, E. Galinsky, and J.E. Swanberg. *The 1997 National Study of the Changing Workforce*. New York: Families and Work Institute, 1998.
10. See Note 5
11. Ibid
12. Ibid

13. *Valuing the Invaluable: The Economic Value of Family Caregiving, 2008 Update.* AARP Public Policy Institute. Retrieved March 13, 2009 from http://assets.aarp.org/rgcenter/il/i13_caregiving.pdf.

14. Family Caregiver Alliance website – www.Caregiver.org. Statistics and Demographics. Retrieved September 29, 2007.

15. Personal Communications with Gary Barg via e-mail received on October 28, 2008.

16. Definition of Suzanne Mintz, co-founder and president of the National Family Caregivers Association - www.NFCAcares.org.

17. J.A. Foreman. *A Web of Information Untangled.* The Boston Globe. Retrieved November 28, 2005 from www.boston.com/yourlife/health/women/articles/2005/11/28/a_web_of_information_untangled.

18. D. Thompson. *The 'Net: A Tangled Web of Health Information.* Health Day. Retrieved April 24, 2008 from www.healthday.com/Article.asp?AID=611014&emc=el&m=1640175&l=33&v=7cc00a7c1e.

19. S. Shellenbarger. *Wanted: Caregiver for Elderly Woman; Only Family Members Need Apply.* The Wall Street Journal. June 20, 2002. Page D2.

20. Ibid

21. Ibid

22. R.E. Silverman. *Who Will Take Care of Mom? Check her Family Contract.* The Wall Street Journal. September 17, 2006.

23. J. Feder, H.L. Komisar, and R. Friedland. *Long-Term Care Financing: Policy Options for the Future.* Georgetown University. June 2007. Retrieved April 24, 2008 from http://ltc.georgetown.edu/forum/ltcfinalpaper061107.pdf.

24. Centers for Medicare and Medicaid. *Medicare & You 2009.* Page 116. Retrieved March 13, 2009 from www.medicare.gov/Publications/Pubs/pdf/10050.pdf.

25. Nationwide® Insurance – www.nationwide.com.

26. SeniorResource.com ezine. March 2004 Edition. Referencing a 2003 GE Center for Financial Learning Survey.

27. Dad. 1989. www.imdb.com/title/tt0097142.

28. K. Greene. *Are Mom and Dad OK?* The Wall Street Journal. November 17, 2002.

29. *A Profile of Caregiving in America (2005)*. The Pfizer Journal. Retrieved May 3, 2006 from www.hawaii.edu/hivandaids/ A%20Profile%20of%20Caregiving%20in%20America.pdf.

30. *John Hancock Survey Finds Many American Affected By Caregiving For Aging Friends & Family.* PRNewswire-FirstCall. November 16, 2006.

31. *Family Caregivers: What They Spend, What They Sacrifice.* National Alliance for Caregiving and Evercare. Retrieved August 11, 2008 from www.caregiving.org/data/Evercare_NAC_CaregiverCostStudyFINA L20111907.pdf.

32. *So Far Away: Twenty Questions for Long-Distance Caregivers.* National Institute on Aging. Retrieved January 28, 2009 from www.nia.nih.gov/HealthInformation/Publications/LongDistanceCa regiving.

33. Driving Miss Daisy. 1989. www.imdb.com/title/tt0097239.

34. *Take Care of Yourself*. Alzheimer's Association. Retrieved February 27, 2004 from www.alz.org/national/documents/brochure_caregiverstress.pdf.

35. *Caregiver Burden and Widower Effect: Elderly's Risk of Death Substantially Increased When a Spouse is Hospitalized or Dies.* Harvard Medical School. Retrieved October 9, 2008 from www.hcp.med.harvard.edu/node/1471.

36. The Caregiver's Bill of Rights. http://catholiccharitiesswo.org/programs/caregiver.html.

37. J. Johnson. *Heartbreaking Work*. The Wall Street Journal. February 17, 2008.

38. Ibid

39. S. E. Merkerson. *The Continuing Journey of a Caregiver*. Cure Magazine. Spring 2003. Page 80.

40. R. Browning. http://poetry.about.com/od/poems/l/blbrowningbenezra.htm.

41. Conversation with Dr. Evelyn Fitzwater, Associate Director of the Center for Aging with Dignity at the University of Cincinnati College of Nursing and professor of Gerontology.

42. Hayflick limit - http://en.wikipedia.org/wiki/Hayflick_limit

43. *A Profile of Older Americans 2008.* Administration on Aging. Retrieved January 28, 2009 from www.aoa.gov/AoAroot/Aging_Statistics/Profile/2008/index.aspx.

44. Centers for Disease Prevention and Control, National Center for Health Statistics, *Preventing the Diseases of Aging*, Volume 12, Number 3, Fall 1999. Retrieved November 28, 2005 from www.cdc.gov/nccdphp/publications/cdnr/pdf/cdfall99.pdf

45. Centers for Disease Prevention and Control, National Center for Health Statistics. Retrieved August 20, 2009 from http://cdc.gov/media/pressrel/2009/r090819.htm (press release), www.cdc.gov/nchs/data/nvsr/nvsr58/nvsr58_01.pdf (full report).

46. R. Winslow. *Yes, You Can Turn Back the Clock.* The Wall Street Journal. May, 18, 2002. Page D1.

47. S. Eder. *Worried about getting older? Forget about it and be happy.* The Cincinnati Enquirer. July, 31, 2002. Page A1.

48. K. Douglas. *What Old Age Taught Me.* Newsweek. August 11, 2008. Page 20.

49. J. Bryner. *Aging just a number: Elderly feel 13 years younger. What Old Age Taught Me.* Retrieved December 4, 2008 from www.msnbc.msn.com/id/28056053.

50. E.A. Phelan and E.B. Larson. *"Successful Aging" – Where Next?* Journal of the American Geriatrics Society., 50(7):1306-1308, 2002.

51. E.A. Phelan, L.A. Anderson, A.Z. Lacroix, and E.B. Larson. *Older Adults' Views of "Successful Aging" – How Do They Compare with Researchers' Definitions?* Journal of the American Geriatrics Society. 52(2):211-216. 2004.

52. Stein Institute at University of California San Diego - http://sira.ucsd.edu.

53. *Scientists Warn Against Anti-Aging Hype.* Science Daily. Retrieved May 21, 2002 from www.sciencedaily.com/releases/2002/05/020521071320.htm.

54. C. Arnst. *Aging Is Becoming So Yesterday".* Business Week. October 11, 2004.

55. See reference 43.

56. S. Carpenter. *Treating an Illness Is One Thing. What About a Patient With Many?* New York Times. Retrieved March 30, 2009 from

www.nytimes.com/2009/03/31/health/31sick.html?_r=1&scp=16
&sq=elderly&st=cse).

57. A.M. Dellinger and J.A. Stevens. *The Injury Problem Among Older Adults: Mortality, Morbidity and Costs.* Journal of Safety Research. 37, 519-522. 2006.

58. *The State of Aging and Health in America 2007 Report.* Centers for Disease Control and Prevention. Retrieved January 28, 2009 from www.cdc.gov/aging/pdf/saha_2007.pdf.

59. J.W. Long. *The Essential Guide to Chronic Illness.* Harper Perennial. New York. 1997.
http://openlibrary.org/b/OL1007814M/essential_
_guide_to_chronic_illness

60. See reference 43.

61. Ibid

62. Learning Pyramid. National Training Laboratories. Bethel, Maine.

63. See reference 43.

64. S. Brink. *Getting on with life after a heart attack.* The Los Angeles Times. October 29, 2007. Page F1.

65. CDC Fact Sheet. Retrieved January 28, 2009 from www.cdc.gov/nccdphp/dnpa/physical/pdf/lifestyles.pdf.

66. R.L. Hotz. *Secrets of the "Wellderly".* The Wall Street Journal. September 19, 2008. Page A18.

67. *Beyond Health Care: New Directions to a Healthier America.* Robert Wood Johnson Foundation. Retrieved April 2, 2009 from www.commissiononhealth.org/NewsRelease.aspx?news=68383.

68. Ibid

69. A.G. Lueckenotte and M. Wallace, M. (2000) *Gerontologic Nursing* (2nd ed., pp. 217-222). St. Louis, MO: Mosby.

70. C.A. Miller. (2003) *Nursing for Wellness in Older Adults* (4th ed., pp. 123-137). Philadelphia, PA: Lippincott Willams & Wilkins.

71. CDC Fact Sheet – 2008.

72. Bill Hettler. The Past of Wellness.
http://hettler.com/History/hettler.htm.

73. B. Spencer. *The Art of Aging Well.* Creative Living. Summer 2002. Pages 19-22.

74. *What is your greatest fear about retirement?* USA Today Snapshots®. April 25, 2005.

75. *Our greatest fears about getting old.* USA Today Snapshots®. February 28, 2006.

76. *Families of Chronically Ill Patients.* Course #9168. Release Date June 1, 2007. CME Resource. Sacramento, CA. www.NetCE.com.

77. L. J. Phillips. *(2006) Dropping the Bomb: The experience of Being Diagnosed with Parkinson's Disease.* Geriatric Nursing, 27(6).

78. Personal interview with Stroke survivor on April 12, 2009.

79. Personal interview with a patient at an acute care hospital in Cincinnati August 24, 2006.

80. D. Grady. *Cancer Patients, Lost in a Maze of Uneven Care.* The New York Times. July 29, 2007.

81. R. Pennebaker. *Having Cancer, and Finding a Personality.* New York Times. August 12, 2008.

82. P. Bronson. *Dignity, ability: That's beautiful.* The Cincinnati Enquirer. May 5, 2005.

83. J. Zaslow. *Another Agony of Alzheimer's: Deciding How – and When – to Say: "I Have It..'* The Wall Street Journal. August 22, 2002.

84. Ibid.

85. See reference 77

86. See reference 76

87. E.J. Taylor, P. Jones, and M. Burns. *Quality of Life.* In I.M. Lubkin and P.D. Larsen (eds.) Chronic Illness: Impact and Interventions. Massachusetts: Jones and Bartlett Publishers. 1998.

88. M. Curtin, I Lubkin. *What is Chronicity?* In I.M. Lubkin and P.D. Larsen (eds.) Chronic Illness: Impact and Interventions. Massachusetts: Jones and Bartlett Publishers. 1998. 3-25. 50.

89. See reference 87.

90. T.A. Rando. (1992). *The Increasing Prevalence of Complicated Mourning: The Onslaught Is Just Beginning.* Omega: Journal of Death and Dying. 26(1):43-59. 49.

91. N.L. Sidell. (1997) *Adult Adjustment to Chronic Illness: A Review of the Literature.* Health and Social Work. 22(1):5-11. 71.

92. H. Livneh and R.F. Antonak. (2005) *Psychosocial Adaptation to Chronic Illness and Disability: A Primer for Counselors.* Journal of Counseling & Development. 83(1):12-20.

93. See reference 91.

94. C.S. Roberts, L. Piper, J. Denny, and G. Cuddeback. (1997) *A support group intervention to facilitate young adults' adjustment to cancer.* Health & Social Work. 22(2):133-141.

95. D. Biordi D. *Social Isolation.* In I.M. Lubkin and P.D. Larsen (eds.) Chronic Illness: Impact and Interventions. Massachusetts: Jones and Bartlett Publishers. 1998. 181-203.

96. See reference 49.

97. *Dad's Alzheimer Diagnosis is Meet by Angry Siblings' Denial.* Dear Abby column. January 20, 2004. www.uexpress.com/dearabby/?uc_full_date=20040120.

98. Alzheimer's often confused with aging. USA Today Snapshots®. June 23, 2004.

99. *Fixing to stay: A national survey on housing and home modification issues* - Executive summary. AARP. Washington DC. 2000.

100. US Senate Special Committee on Aging.

101. *2008 Alzheimer's Disease Facts and Figures.* Alzheimer's Association. www.alz.org/national/documents/report_alzfactsfigures2008.pdf.

102. G. Tasker. *Addictions tarnish the golden years.* The Cincinnati Enquirer. November 12, 2003.

103. *Taking the Aches Out of Aging.* The Wall Street Journal. May 9, 2002.

104. F.X. Donnelly and K. Bouffard. *Old, infirmed turn to children.* The Cincinnati Enquirer. February 10, 2004.

105. See reference 43.

106. Ibid.

107. *Enabling: Let Go and Let God.* Living Free Every Day. Daily Devotional from April 15, 2009. http://LivingFree.org.

108. Wikipedia. http://en.wikipedia.org/wiki/Codependent.

109. A. Kron. *Meeting the Challenge: Living with Chronic Illness.* www.ChronicIllness.com.

110. J.A. Romas, and M. Sharma. *Practical stress management. A comprehensive workbook for promoting health and managing change through* stress reduction. (5th ed.). San Francisco, CA: Benjamin Cummings. Page 77.

111. J. Leland. *In 'Sweetie' and 'Dear,' a Hurt for the Elderly.* The New York Times. Retrieved November 6, 2008 from www.nytimes.com/2008/10/07/us/07aging.html?_r=2.

112. E. H. F. Law http://missionfunding.pcusa.org/peacemaking/iraq/biblestudies.htm

113. *Seniors Fear Loss of Independence, Nursing Homes More Than Death.* November 12, 2007. Retrieved August 28, 2009 from www.marketing charts.com/direct/seniors-fear-loss-of-independence-nursing-homes-more-than-death-2343.

114. S. Classen, S. Winter, and E.D.S. Lopez. *(2009) Meta-synthesis of Qualitative Studies on Older Driver Safety and Mobility.* Occupation, Participation and Health. 29(1). pp 24-31.

115. S. Sabalos. *Oh, grow up!* The Cincinnati Enquirer. Date unknown.

116. L. Green and M. Kreuter PRECEED-PROCEED Model. www.comminit.com/en/node/27126/36

117. C.A. Bruce. (2002). *The grief process for patient, family and physician.* Journal of the American Osteopathic Association. Supplement 3, Vol. 102, No. 9, S28-S32.

118. Ibid.

119. Ibid.

120. J. Eldridge. (2001) *Wild At Heart.* Thomas Nelson. Nashville, TN. www.ransomedheart.com.

121. C.W. Metcalf, and R. Felible, R. (1992). *Lightening Up: Survival Skills for People Under Pressure.* Cambridge, Mass: Perseus Books.

122. Kubler-Ross Model. http://en.wikipedia.org/wiki/K%C3%BCbler-Ross_model.

123. I. Maddocks. (2003) *Grief and bereavement,* Medical Journal of Australia, Supplement 6, Vol. 179, S6-S7.

124. See reference 116.

125. Chaplin D. Lewis. Editorial. Loveland Herald. November 19, 2003.

126. W.H Beebe. Death and The City. The New York Times. January 17, 2004.

127. *Nursing Home Visitors are Encouraged to Lend a Hand.* Dear Abby column. June 20, 2002. www.uexpress.com/dearabby/?uc_full_date=20020620.